Noninvasive Techniques for Assessment of Atherosclerosis
in Peripheral, Carotid, and Coronary Arteries

Noninvasive Techniques for Assessment of Atherosclerosis in Peripheral, Carotid, and Coronary Arteries

Editors

Thomas F. Budinger, M.D., Ph.D.
Henry Miller Professor of Research Medicine
Donner Laboratory
University of California
Berkeley, California

Alan S. Berson, Ph.D.
Devices and Technology Branch
National Heart, Lung, and Blood Institute
National Institutes of Health
Bethesda, Maryland

Ivar Ringqvist, M.D.
Cardiac Diseases Branch
National Heart, Lung, and Blood Institute
National Institutes of Health
Bethesda, Maryland

Michael B. Mock, M.D.
Chief, Cardiac Diseases Branch
National Heart, Lung, and Blood Institute
National Institutes of Health
Bethesda, Maryland

John T. Watson, Ph.D.
Chief, Devices and Technology Branch
National Heart, Lung, and Blood Institute
National Institutes of Health
Bethesda, Maryland

Roger S. Powell
Devices and Technology Branch
National Heart, Lung and Blood Institute
National Institutes of Health
Bethesda, Maryland

Raven Press ■ New York

Raven Press, 1140 Avenue of the Americas, New York, New York 10036

Made in the United States of America

International Standard Book Number 0-89004-679-4
Library of Congress Catalog Number 81-40614

Foreword

This volume on the noninvasive assessment of cardiovascular disease is an important undertaking. It is impossible to overemphasize the magnitude of the atherosclerosis problem.

Atherosclerosis will be responsible for 85% of the cardiovascular deaths in the United States this year, is primarily responsible for 1 1/2 million heart attacks and more than 500,000 strokes annually. The disease is thought to cost us more than $50 billion each year and its sequelae are the primary causes of disability under the Social Security system in this country.

Atherosclerosis is a silent disease; we cannot determine its extent in any individual or vascular tree until it produces signs or symptoms through occlusion or embolism. As much as two-thirds of the coronary lumen may be occluded by atherosclerotic plaque without any signs or symptoms. Suddenly, we see with further occlusion or vasospasm symptomatic disease manifested by chest pain, heart attack, or sudden death. Since the first sign of atherosclerosis is often the last sign, we cannot afford to aim our therapy at symptomatic cardiovascular disease only.

Cardiovascular epidemiologists have spent the past 20 to 30 years defining cardiovascular risk factors—predisposing early traits or habits. Cardiovascular physiologists have taken another equally important tack. Using several new techniques, they have sought to document the atherosclerotic process by trying to visualize the vascular system and blood flow throughout, long before signs or symptoms of disease appear.

The ability to view the large and small vessels in an individual and to record within millimeters the amount of atherosclerotic plaque would greatly aid in diagnosis. With an assurance based on data obtained without apparent risk to the patient, a physician could discuss the prognosis of an individual who may appear well but who exhibits the risk factors of atherosclerosis. One could then detect disease before damage becomes irreversible—one could diagnose coronary disease before heart attacks occur.

Perhaps the greatest promise of noninvasive technology is its potential for shortening the expensive, lengthy clinical trials in atherosclerosis, which require definite results, such as heart attack and death. It is heartening to think that we may be able to evaluate new therapies of all forms without requiring such morbid results that take a long time to develop.

These are not new concepts. In the early 1970s the Atherosclerosis Task Force and the Advisory Council stressed the need for further development of noninvasive techniques. The National Heart, Lung, and Blood Institute developed a contract program to begin work on noninvasive techniques as a specific, solicited target area for 1975 and continued the program in 1977. We supported contracts both under and outside the solicitation, aiming to move the field along as rapidly as possible.

Much of our investment thus far has been in ultrasound techniques, but we have also supported X-ray image intensification and one project on the use of nuclear magnetic resonance.

We would like to see what we have, where we are, and what the limits are on what we can and expect to do. We would like to define where we can go and what we can expect over the next 5 to 10 years. Of course, the issue of resources may prevent us from getting where we would like to be, but that is secondary.

The first issue is to determine what is possible and practical in this area. We appear to be at a crossroad and we may be ready to begin validating noninvasive techniques, comparing them to the older invasive techniques for assessing lesions in the peripheral vessels. At the same time, it appears that for the smaller interior vessels, like the coronaries, we still await further technical developments.

Robert I. Levy

Preface

This volume has as its objective a review of the state of the art, and the potentials and limitations of noninvasive techniques for detecting, quantifying, and characterizing atherosclerotic lesions in arteries. The material in this monograph provides descriptions of the clinical needs, present instrumentation, validation techniques, and future research opportunities in this area. The scientists whose work is represented here have contributed to advances in this field. They represent the disciplines of cardiology, epidemiology, biostatistics, bioengineering, physics, physiology, pathology, radiology, computer processing, and surgery that have converged to produce these advancements. Each of the chapters is written so as to be independently comprehensible to the reader who is somewhat knowledgeable in one or more of these areas.

The major noninvasive techniques of ultrasound, X-ray, nuclear medicine, positron emission, and nuclear magnetic resonance are discussed in depth in various chapters. Readers who may be only casually interested in this area of cardiovascular diagnosis will find valuable review and overview material in some chapters. Other chapters deal in considerable depth with technical and scientific aspects that will be of special interest to researchers and clinicians who are working directly in this area.

Alan S. Berson

Acknowledgment

This monograph is based upon a Workshop, sponsored by the National Heart, Lung, and Blood Institute, Bethesda, Maryland. The Workshop Chairperson was Richard S. Ross. Co-chairpersons were Thomas F. Budinger, Bernadine H. Bulkley, James E. Dalen, and Colin J. Schwartz.

Contents

Present Noninvasive Methods: State of the Art, Limitations, and Potential Capabilities

Contributors

M. Arakawa
Radiologic Imaging Laboratory
University of California
South San Francisco, California 94080

D. W. Baker
Advanced Technology Laboratories
2100 124th Avenue, NE
Bellevue, Washington 98005

M. R. Ball
Bowman Gray School of Medicine
Wake Forest University
Winston-Salem, North Carolina 27103

R. W. Barnes
Department of Surgery
Medical College of Virginia
Virginia Commonwealth University
Richmond, Virginia 23298

H. Berkoff
Department of Radiology
Clinical Science Center
University of Wisconsin
Madison, Wisconsin 53792

M. G. Bond
Department of Comparative Medicine
Bowman Gray School of Medicine
Wake Forest University
Winston-Salem, North Carolina 27103

T. F. Budinger
Department of Research Medicine
Donner Laboratory
University of California
Berkeley, California 94720

M. P. Capp
Department of Radiology
University of Arizona Health Sciences
Center
Tucson, Arizona 85721

P. L. Carson
Department of Radiology
University of Michigan Hospitals and
Medical School
Ann Arbor, Michigan 48109

P. M. Chikos
Department of Surgery
University of Washington School of
Medicine
Seattle, Washington 98105

P. C. Christenson
Department of Radiology
University of Arizona Health Sciences
Center
Tucson, Arizona 85721

D. W. Crawford
Department of Cardiology
University of Southern California
Los Angeles, California 90033

L. Crooks
Radiologic Imaging Laboratory
University of California
South San Francisco, California 94080

A. B. Crummy
Department of Radiology
Clinical Science Center
University of Wisconsin
Madison, Wisconsin 53792

A. S. Daoud
Department of Pathology
Albany Medical Center
Albany, New York 12208

C. E. Davis
Department of Biostatistics
University of Washington
Seattle, Washington 98105

D. L. Davis
Institute of Applied Physiology and
Medicine
Seattle, Washington 98122

H. T. Dodge
Department of Medicine
Division of Cardiology
University of Washington
Seattle, Washington 98105

J. E. Edwards
Department of Pathology
United Hospitals
St. Paul, Minnesota 55102

D. E. Ergun
Department of Radiology
Clinical Science Center
University of Wisconsin
Madison, Wisconsin 53792

T. C. Evans, Jr.
Cardiovascular Division
Mayo Foundation
Mayo Medical School
Rochester, Minnesota 55901

H. D. Fisher III
Department of Radiology
University of Arizona Health Sciences
 Center
Tucson, Arizona 85721

L. Fisher
Department of Surgery
University of Washington School of
 Medicine
Seattle, Washington 98105

K. E. Fritz
Albany Medical Center
Albany, New York 12208

M. M. Frost
Department of Radiology
University of Arizona Health Sciences
 Center
Tucson, Arizona 85721

S. Glagov
Department of Pathology
University of Chicago
Chicago, Illinois 60637

K. L. Gould
Division of Cardiology
University of Texas Medical School
Houston, Texas 77025

J. F. Greenleaf
Department of Biophysics and Medicine
Mayo Foundation
Mayo Medical School
Rochester, Minnesota 55901

W. R. Harlan
Department of Postgraduate Medicine
Health Professions Education
University of Michigan
Ann Arbor, Michigan 48109

L. D. Harris
Mayo Foundation
Mayo Medical School
Rochester, Minnesota 55901

R. Herfkens
Radiologic Imaging Laboratory
University of California
South San Francisco, California 94080

J. H. Hirsch
Department of Surgery
University of Washington School of
 Medicine
Seattle, Washington 98105

J. Hoenninger
Radiologic Imaging Laboratory
University of California
South San Francisco, California 94080

D. I. Hoult
Biomedical Engineering and
 Instrumentation Branch
Division of Research Services
National Institutes of Health
Bethesda, Maryland 20205

J. Jarmolych
Albany Medical Center
Albany, New York 12208

M. P. Judkins
Department of Radiology
Loma Linda University Medical Center
Loma Linda, California 92350

J. M. Kaduck
Bowman Gray School of Medicine
Wake Forest University
Winston-Salem, North Carolina 27103

A. S. Katocs, Jr.
Department of Biology
Medical Research Division
American Cyanamid Company
Pearl River, New York 10965

L. Kaufman
Radiologic Imaging Laboratory
University of California
South San Francisco, California 94080

R. A. Kruger
Department of Radiology
Clinical Science Center
University of Wisconsin
Madison, Wisconsin 53792

J. R. Landis
Department of Postgraduate Medicine
Health Professions Education
University of Michigan
Ann Arbor, Michigan 48109

P. C. Lauterbur
Department of Chemistry
State University of New York at Stony
Brook
Stony Brook, New York 11794

R. I. Levy
School of Medicine
Tufts University
Boston, Massachusetts 02111

G. C. McMillan
Atherosclerosis, Hypertension, and Lipid
Metabolism Section
Division of Heart and Vascular Diseases
National Heart, Lung, and Blood
Institute
National Institutes of Health
Bethesda, Maryland 20205

R. McRee
Radiologic Imaging Laboratory
University of California
South San Francisco, California 94080

A. F. Metherell
Department of Radiology
South Bay Hospital
Redondo Beach, California 90277

C. A. Mistretta
Department of Radiology
Clinical Science Center
University of Wisconsin
Madison, Wisconsin 53792

D. Myerowitz
Department of Radiology
Clinical Science Center
University of Wisconsin
Madison, Wisconsin 53792

S. Nudelman
Department of Radiology
University of Arizona Health Sciences
Center
Tucson, Arizona 85721

W. H. Oldendorf
Department of Neurology
School of Medicine
University of California at Los Angeles
Los Angeles, California 90024

T. W. Ovitt
Department of Radiology
University of Arizona Health Sciences
Center
Tucson, Arizona 85721

J. M. Reid
Department of Bioengineering
Institute of Applied Physiology and
Medicine
Seattle, Washington 98122

W. A. Riley
Bowman Gray School of Medicine
Wake Forest University
Winston-Salem, North Carolina 27103

E. L. Ritman
Department of Physiology and Medicine
Biodynamics Research Unit
Mayo Foundation
Rochester, Minnesota 55901

H. Roehrig
Department of Radiology
University of Arizona Health Sciences
Center
Tucson, Arizona 85721

R. S. Ross
Department of Medicine
Johns Hopkins University School of
Medicine
Baltimore, Maryland 21218

J. F. Sackett
Department of Radiology
Clinical Science Center
University of Wisconsin
Madison, Wisconsin 53792

T. M. Sapp
Department of Biology
Medical Research Division
American Cyanamid Company
Pearl River, New York 10965

S. A. Schaffer
Department of Biology
Medical Research Division
American Cyanamid Company
Pearl River, New York 10965

G. Seeley
Department of Radiology
University of Arizona Health Sciences
* Center*
Tucson, Arizona 85721

R. H. Selzer
Biomedical Image Processing Laboratory
Jet Propulsion Laboratory
California Institute of Technology
Pasadena, California 91109

C. G. Shaw
Department of Radiology
Clinical Science Center
University of Wisconsin
Madison, Wisconsin 53792

M. P. Spencer
Institute of Applied Physiology and
* Medicine*
Seattle, Washington 98122

D. E. Strandness, Jr.
Department of Surgery
University of Washington School of
* Medicine*
Seattle, Washington 98195

H. W. Strauss
Nuclear Medicine Division
Massachusetts General Hospital
Boston, Massachusetts 02114

C. Strother
Department of Radiology
Clinical Science Center
University of Wisconsin
Madison, Wisconsin 53792

D. S. Sumner
Department of Surgery
Section of Peripheral Vascular Surgery
Southern Illinois University School of
* Medicine*
St. John's Hospital
Springfield, Illinois 62769

B. L. Thiele
Department of Surgery
University of Washington School of
* Medicine*
Seattle, Washington 98195

W. A. Thomas
Albany Medical Center
Albany, New York 12208

J. F. Toole
Department of Neurology
Bowman Gray School of Medicine
Wake Forest University
Winston-Salem, North Carolina 27103

W. Turnipseed
Department of Radiology
Clinical Science Center
University of Wisconsin
Madison, Wisconsin 53792

M. Van Lysel
Department of Radiology
Clinical Science Center
University of Wisconsin
Madison, Wisconsin 53792

J. Watts
Radiologic Imaging Laboratory
University of California
South San Francisco, California 94080

P. N. T. Wells
Department of Medical Physics
Bristol General Hospital
Bristol, BS1 65Y United Kingdom

A. E. Weyman
Department of Medicine
Indiana University School of Medicine
University Hospital
Indianapolis, Indiana 46202

C. K. Zarins
Department of Surgery
University of Chicago
Chicago, Illinois 60637

W. Zwiebel
Department of Radiology
Clinical Science Center
University of Wisconsin
Madison, Wisconsin 53792

Noninvasive Techniques for Assessment of Atherosclerosis in Peripheral, Carotid, and Coronary Arteries, edited by Thomas F. Budinger, et al. Raven Press, New York 1982.

Introduction

Thomas F. Budinger, Alan S. Berson, Ivar Ringqvist, Michael B. Mock, John T. Watson, and Roger S. Powell

From the earliest times, progress in understanding the pathophysiology of an organ system has been closely related to our ability to study and understand the structure of the organ, both in the normal and diseased state. Recently, dramatic progress has been made in our ability to understand the structure, function, and metabolism of the cardiovascular system and to make precise anatomical diagnoses in patients using noninvasive techniques. The development of many of these techniques has been supported and nurtured by the National Heart, Lung, and Blood Institute (NHLBI) through a variety of support mechanisms, including investigator-initiated grants, special targeted grants, and contract programs. These noninvasive methods are being used with greater frequency and clinical accuracy. Improvements have paralleled and often made possible the remarkable advances in treating cardiovascular disease. Today, in community hospitals and medical clinics across the land, cardiologists use knowledge and diagnostic modalities that did not exist a few years ago.

This monograph will cover the major noninvasive techniques used in the cardiovascular field; the major emphasis will be on the use of imaging techniques to evaluate obstructive plaques occurring in the carotid, femoral, and coronary arteries. Among the techniques discussed are subtraction radiography, X-ray tomography, echocardiography, Doppler ultrasonic flow methods, radioisotopic methods, positron emission transaxial tomography, and nuclear magnetic resonance. Certainly, the noninvasive techniques that are considered have broader applications in the study of structure and function of the cardiovascular system.

Some of the techniques presented are invasive. These "invasive" noninvasive techniques require intravenous injections and include subtraction radiographic and radionuclide studies. They are included in this monograph because they do not require an intraarterial catheter, making the invasiveness considerably less important in terms of morbidity and mortality. There is presently no "ideal" noninvasive diagnostic technique with which to study the cardiovascular system. These techniques are complementary and require continual research and development to improve patient benefit.

One modality not included in this volume is that using microwave frequency interrogation. This technique consists of forming images using non-ionizing electromagnetic radiation in the 10 MHz to 10 GHz frequency range. The characteristics determining the resultant images are tissue dielectric properties and geometry. This technique has not yet been applied toward imaging lesions in arteries, and no formal papers were presented at the NHLBI workshop describing such an approach. However, the workshop participants did discuss the potentials for this technique, concluding that practical applications will need to await major technological advancements.

This monograph covers the field broadly, not only in the range of noninvasive diagnostic techniques available, but also in the cross-section of technical and medical disciplines of those who are involved in the research and clinical application of noninvasive techniques in the diagnosis of cardiovascular disease. It is the goal of this monograph to present the state of the art of these techniques by researchers and clinicians who have made major contributions and developments in this field. Some of the techniques included are already now routinely used, such as echocardiography and Doppler ultrasonic methods. Others, such as dynamic spatial reconstruction (DSR), positron emission transaxial tomography (PETT), and nuclear magnetic resonance (NMR) are currently research tools with very limited clinical applications.

In this introductory chapter, we will present a brief overview of the techniques which are discussed in greater detail in subsequent chapters. Included are the present and future applications, the basic concepts of the techniques, and, when possible, the interrelationships among the different approaches.

SUBTRACTION ANGIOGRAPHY

Although angiocardiography has proven valuable in identifying cardiac structure and function, it is accomplished with some hazard to the patient. The skilled angiographer can usually perform this test with minimal risk to the patient. Often the anatomical and hemodynamic information derived from these techniques is essential for establishing a correct diagnosis and planning a logical therapeutic approach for patient management and thus justifies the risk (1). The complications of angiocardiography have led to a continuing search for less invasive techniques that can be performed with lower risk and dose of radiation or no radiation at all. One of the newer research techniques for evaluating the cardiovascular system by radiography is intravenous angiography using digital video subtraction, sometimes called subtraction angiography.

Subtraction angiography is an application of what can be called photoelectronic radiography because the X-rays which pass through the patient are detected by a sensitive X-ray image intensifier and television camera instead of by radiographic film (2). The image information is then processed by a computer where it is possible to manipulate the image parameters electronically so as to enhance the contrast of a low-contrast image or to subtract out undesirable information from surrounding tissues. With this technique, it is possible to avoid catheterization by injecting a radiopaque contrast agent intravenously, subtract the images before and after injection, and enhance the image contrast to equal that of a conventional arteriogram (Fig. 1). Another method of subtraction radiography involves the subtraction of two images recorded at the same time at two different X-ray energy levels. The resultant image is not confounded by motion artifacts.

Subtraction angiography has potential for evaluating the structure and function of the heart and coronary arteries. This technique may also be valuable in examining

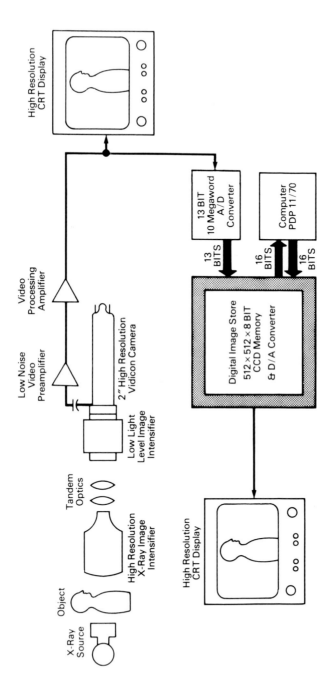

FIG. 1. Flow diagram showing the basic concepts of the X-ray subtraction technique. The X-rays which pass through the patient are detected by an image intensifier and then processed and stored in the computer. The enhanced images can be subsequently viewed on a TV display.

intracranial circulation where ultrasonic imaging and flow measurements cannot yet be applied. Images can also be selectively enlarged. Patients have been successfully examined and diagnosed as outpatients. Therefore, costs are reduced since hospitalization for arteriography is not required and risks are also reduced.

DYNAMIC SPATIAL RECONSTRUCTION

Dynamic spatial reconstruction (DSR) is an X-ray research method that is showing promise for being able to produce three-dimensional images of the cardiovascular system in the intact, living patient (3). With the DSR technique, the patient is positioned in the center of the machine in the field of X-ray tubes and multiple X-ray views are obtained using surrounding X-ray tubes at various levels throughout the body of the patient (Fig. 2). The information is stored in a computer system.

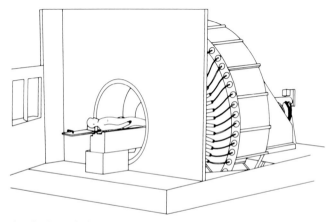

FIG. 2. A patient is shown being positioned in the center of the dynamic spatial reconstruction machine. This unit contains a circular array of X-ray tubes which permits multiple X-ray views which are then reconstructed into volume displays by the computer.

The computer-stored images can be reconstructed for any cross-section through the heart (Fig. 3). The unique feature of the DSR is that it produces volume reconstruction as distinct from the slice reconstruction of commercial computed tomography scanners. This volume imaging permits retrospective selection of appropriate sections through the region of interest. Furthermore, a combination of electronic and mechanical sequencing of the multiple X-ray tubes permits a volume image to be obtained within a short enough period of time to minimize motion artifacts.

ECHOCARDIOGRAPHY

Many of the advantages of noninvasive methods for evaluating anatomy and function of the heart are embodied in the echocardiographic technique. This technique does not require ionizing radiation and has no known risk; therefore, it can be performed repeatedly on patients at any age and at any time in a hospital at the patient's bedside or on an outpatient basis. The principle by which ultrasound creates

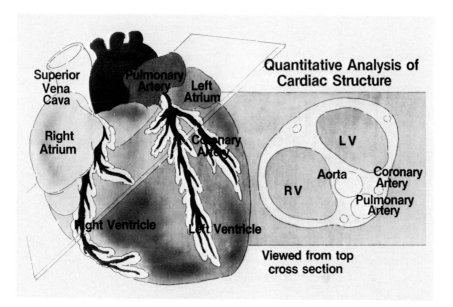

FIG. 3. Computer-stored images can be reconstructed for any cross-section through the heart.

an image is shown in Fig. 4. The transducer is held against the chest wall. It contains a piezoelectric element that vibrates very rapidly and produces ultrasonic pulses or waves. The various structures which the beam transects produce echoes which are reflected back to the chest wall, detected by the transducer, and then processed and displayed on a chart recorder or an oscilloscope. The M-mode echocardiogram produces a one-dimensional image as a function of time. Changing the direction of the ultrasonic beam permits different views of the heart to be obtained, revealing information regarding the internal dimensions, structure, and dynamic function of the heart. M-mode echocardiography was one of the earliest ultrasonic noninvasive techniques developed for cardiovascular examination.

The M-mode echocardiogram can be diagnostic in certain cardiac disorders such as mitral stenosis or idiopathic hypertrophic subaortic stenosis (4). It has proven to be extremely valuable, especially in recording cardiac motion that is perpendicular to the ultrasonic beam.

The major limitations of M-mode scanning are that it does not permit effective evaluation of cardiac shape and it cannot depict lateral motion. This has led to the development of cross-sectional, or two-dimensional, echocardiography often referred to as B-scan (Fig. 4). This technique provides additional information that is not available with the M-mode method. In this technique, the tip of the transducer is held stationary and the transmitting acoustic beam is moved mechanically in an arc by oscillating a single transducer or by rotating a series of transducers. Alternatively, a transducer array may be electronically scanned. Some scanners have hand-held transducers. The operator may translate the acoustic assembly over the area of interest to sweep out an image in which both vertical and horizontal axes are representative of distances along the target tissue. By utilizing this type of ultrasonic technique, we can obtain cross-sectional information about the heart

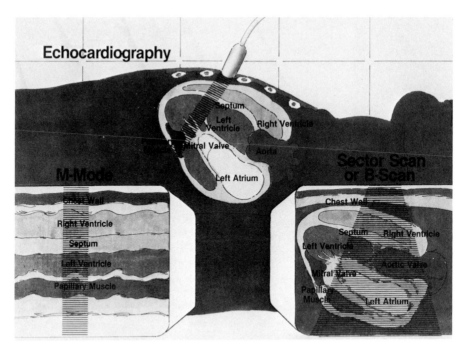

FIG. 4. The principle by which ultrasound waves are produced by a transducer held against the surface of the chest. The M-mode **(left)** is a one-dimensional image as a function of time. The sector or B-scan **(right)** provides a two-dimensional cross-sectional image.

chambers and valves either in the form of a sector view or a rectilinear B-scan (5). The cross-sectional echocardiography technology is still evolving, and factors such as angle of display, frame or sweep line density, image persistence, depth of examination, and beam characteristics are constantly changing and vary among different instruments. The NHLBI continues to support a great deal of basic and applied research in ultrasonic techniques for examination of the heart.

Many disorders of the cardiovascular system that account for a great amount of morbidity and mortality are secondary to lesions in the peripheral or carotid arteries. Most cerebral infarctions are the result of atherosclerosis and, because carotid disease is responsible for almost half of them, the detection of plaques in the carotid arteries during the asymptomatic phase or early in the symptomatic phase of an illness can be extremely important. Angiography of the carotid arteries is now used frequently to evaluate patients presenting with transient ischemic attacks; still, carotid angiography has a significant complication rate. Therefore, there is a need to identify more precisely those patients in whom angiography is indicated. Over 90 percent of carotid plaques lie in the region of the carotid bifurcation where they can be assessed by noninvasive methods of detection. Ultrasonic B-scan techniques have been shown to be effective tools for identification of obstructive plaques in these arteries and in peripheral arteries of the extremities. Both longitudinal and transverse images of arterial lumens may be obtained. A subtle, but important, distinction between ultrasonic and X-ray techniques is that the former images arterial wall and plaque, whereas the lumen carrying contrast agent is imaged by X-ray. The ultrasonic method thus has a potential for characterizing plaque composition based upon acoustic properties of different types of plaque. Future research may be directed towards developing this potential.

DOPPLER TECHNIQUE

With the Doppler technique, ultrasonic waves are reflected from a moving object such as the formed elements in a column of blood. The frequency of the received signal is different from that of the transmitted signal. This difference depends on the velocity of the reflecting interface and the angle at which the beam strikes the object; this is frequently referred to as the "Doppler shift." When Doppler ultrasound is used to examine the velocity of blood flow, the ultrasonic energy is reflected by the blood cells and platelets. This application of ultrasound has been used primarily to evaluate blood flow in superficial peripheral vessels such as carotid arteries and veins. It has also proven useful in detecting obstructions in deeper peripheral arteries and in detecting thrombosis in the deeper peripheral veins. Recent advanced Doppler instruments, called duplex systems, combine the Doppler mode with the B-scan ultrasound mode, making it possible to have both an image of the vessel wall and lesions and additional information on the magnitude and direction of blood flow (6).

Figure 5 depicts the basic principle of the Doppler technique and illustrates the type of image that can be reconstructed from flow measurements in an artery.

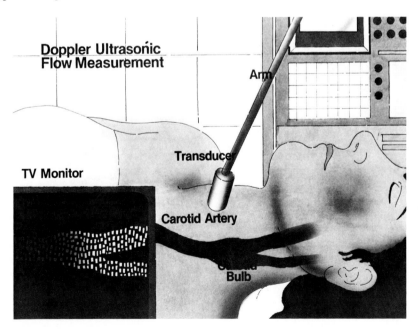

FIG. 5. The principle of Doppler imaging-flow technique, illustrating the transducer and the image that is obtained.

RADIOISOTOPE METHODS

The pioneering work in radionuclides was begun as early as 1927 by Drs. Blum-gard and White using radon gas to study patients with heart disease. Modern radionuclide studies fall into three major classifications: (a) ventricular function studies which are used for measuring cardiac output and providing information on ventricular wall performance; (b) myocardial blood flow or perfusion studies which evaluate blood flow within the myocardium; and (c) myocardial infarction localizing studies for estimating the location and size of certain infarctions (7). Development of the gated blood pool scan technique enabled collection of images during specific portions of the cardiac cycle, that is, during diastole or the filling phase, and during systole or the ejection phase. In this process, the ECG is used to trigger the timing circuits to collect images during systole and diastole. The computer stores these multiple images, and they can later be recalled for viewing (Fig. 6). By collecting

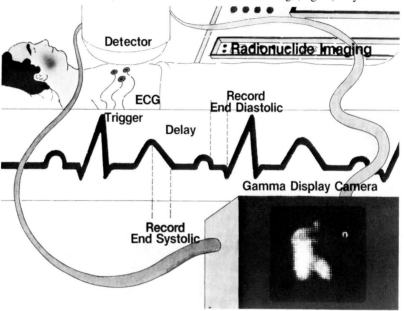

FIG. 6. The principle of the gated radionuclide imaging technique. In this procedure, the ECG is used to trigger timing circuits which permits collection of images at end systole and end diastole. In the righthand corner an image of end systole is shown.

a large number of images of the heart obtained in systole and diastole, the computer can be programmed to display the images sequentially in a manner which resembles the types of cine images obtained by angiocardiography. Thus, the technique has been called radionuclide cineangiography. Radionuclide cine studies can be performed at rest and during exercise, usually by having the patient pedal an inverted bicycle attached above a special table equipped with hand grips to prevent excessive chest motion during exercise.

Another major application of radionuclide techniques in cardiovascular diagnosis is to evaluate regional blood flow in the heart muscle. This application is commonly referred to as a perfusion scan. The most logical decisions regarding surgical or medical treatment for coronary artery disease can be made when there is an objective measurement of regional myocardial blood perfusion. Coronary angiography can illustrate an obstruction in a coronary artery, but it cannot show the effect of this obstruction on tissue perfusion. Myocardial perfusion radionuclide techniques can provide regional myocardial perfusion information.

A third application of radionuclide techniques is in studying acute myocardial infarction. Myocardial scintigrams have been used to diagnose, localize, and determine the size of an acute myocardial infarction. Technetium-99m-pyrophosphate or thalium-201 is used for imaging acute myocardial infarctions.

Some of the current problems associated with conventional radionuclide techniques are overcome with radionuclide tomography which produces two-dimensional reconstructions using positron emitters with short half-lives. In this technique, positron-emitting radionuclide-labeled substances are injected intravenously and are quickly incorporated into the myocardial tissue. The annihilation photons emitted by the isotope are then detected by the circular array of multiple coincidence scintillation crystal detectors surrounding the patient as shown in Fig. 7. This figure

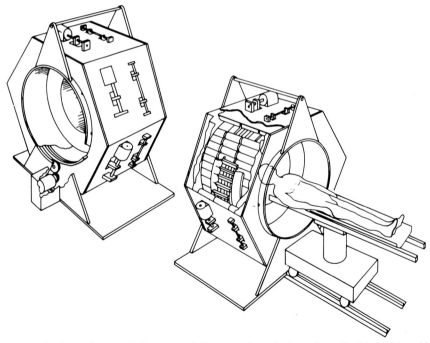

FIG. 7. In the positron emission transaxial tomography technique, the patient is positioned in the center of a machine which contains a circular array of multiple coincidence gamma dectors.

illustrates the PETT scanner developed at Washington University at St. Louis under NHLBI support (8). This is a research technique which is most useful in studying the metabolic turnover of labeled compounds. These labeled compounds with very short half-lives, usually under one hour, must be produced by a cyclotron or linear accelerator on site. The data are processed by a computer and reconstructed into an image representing the distribution of the isotope within the heart. PETT scanning has been applied to the study of ischemic heart disease in man using fatty acids labeled with carbon-11 palmitate (8). Tomography in normal subjects in whom this compound was injected shows a uniform distribution of the carbon-11 palmitate throughout the left ventricle. On the other hand, in patients with a myocardial infarction, the infarcted area fails to show activity.

NUCLEAR MAGNETIC RESONANCE IMAGING

Nuclear magnetic resonance (NMR) imaging is an interesting new development in noninvasive cardiac diagnosis which uses magnetic fields to scan the body from the outside and to reconstruct a cross-sectional image of the anatomy or an image of blood flow patterns (9, 10). The patient is placed in the center of a system of magnetic fields (Fig. 8). A low level radiofrequency (RF) pulse is superimposed.

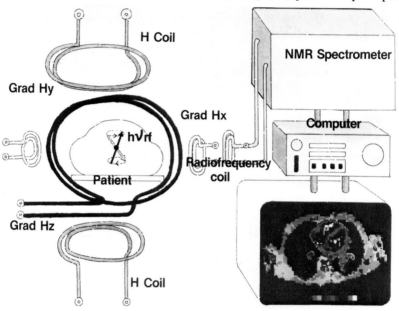

FIG. 8. In the nuclear magnetic resonance technique, the patient is placed in the center of a system of magnetic fields. The radiofrequency coil is energized to superimpose a RF field over the area of interest. Information is obtained about each part in the body under conditions of nuclear magnetic resonance.

Spatial information is obtained by varying the magnetic field distribution or the RF frequency (cf. Crooks et al., *this volume*). As different areas of the body are interrogated by the RF field, different images may be processed by a computer and displayed as a color-coded cross-sectional image of the entire body or portion of the body immersed in the magnetic field.

These images can now be made with resolutions on the order of 2 mm in a fraction of a minute and have no known hazards for the patient, who is not exposed to ionizing radiation. At the present time, NMR is a research tool. Since this technique is based on the magnetic properties of specific atoms in the cells, in the future it might be refined to reveal not only the shape of a cardiac structure or the size of a vessel, but also the tissue composition.

As we look to the future, the ideal noninvasive diagnostic instrument for cardiovascular disease should show us the location and size of the obstructing plaque in an artery and reveal its composition and biological behavior. These ideal instruments should be able to identify whether the thickened wall of the ventricle is secondary to muscle hypertrophy or to infiltration of fibrous or fatty tissue. Each noninvasive modality has strengths and weaknesses, and it is likely that they will be found to have complementary benefits in medical diagnosis.

REFERENCES

1. Davis, K., Kennedy, W., Kemp, H., et al. (1979): Complications of coronary arteriography from the Collaborative Study of Coronary Artery Surgery (CASS). *Circulation*, 59:1105.
2. Ovitt, T. W., Christenson, P. C., Fisher, H. D., Frost, M. M., Nudelman, S., Roehrig, H., Sealey, G. (1980): Intravenous angiography using digital video subtraction: X-ray imaging system and intravenous cervical cerebral vascular angiography. *Am. J. Radiol.*, 135:1141–1152.
3. Ritman, E. L., Robb, R. A., Johnson, S. A., et al. (1978): Quantitative imaging of the structure and function of the heart, lungs, and circulation. *Mayo Clin. Proc.*, 53:3.
4. Feigenbaum, H. (1976): *Echocardiography*, 2nd Edition. Lea & Febiger, Philadelphia.
5. Tajik, A. J., Seward, J. B., Hayler, D. J., et al. (1978): Two-dimensional real-time ultrasound imaging of the heart and great vessels. *Mayo Clin. Proc.*, 53:271.
6. Baker, D. W., Rubenstein, S. A., Lorch, G. S. (1977): Pulsed Doppler echocardiography: Principles and applications. *Am. J. Med.*, 63:69.
7. Strauss, H. W., Pitt, B. (1979): *Cardiovascular Nuclear Medicine*, 2nd Edition, C. V. Mosby, St. Louis.
8. Sobel, B. E., Weiss, E. S., Welch, M. J., Siegel, B. A., and Ter-Pogossian, M. M. (1977): Detection of remote myocardial infarction in patients with positron emission trans-axial tomography and intravenous C-palmitate. *Circulation*, 55:853.
9. Sutherland, R. J., Hutchison, J. M. S. (1978): Three-dimensional NMR imaging using selective excitation. *J. Physical Eng. Sci. Instr.*, II:79–83.
10. Lauterbur, P. C. (1973): Image formation by induced local interactions: examples employing nuclear magnetic resonance. *Nature (London)*, 242:190.

Noninvasive Techniques for Assessment of Atherosclerosis in Peripheral, Carotid, and Coronary Arteries, edited by Thomas F. Budinger, et al. Raven Press, New York 1982.

Atherosclerotic Lesions: Their Distribution and Histopathology

Jesse E. Edwards

Department of Pathology, United Hospitals, St. Paul, Minnesota 55102

This chapter discusses primarily the structural nature and distribution of established atheromatous lesions. Atherosclerosis is a focal process (1), although multiple foci may be involved in a given arterial system. Segments of a normal artery are characteristically found between diseased segments of varying degrees of severity. The focal nature of atherosclerosis may be shown by the histologic appearance of involved segments: One arc of the artery is frequently uninvolved while the remainder contains an atheroma.

ATHEROMA

Various intimal changes cause the lesion commonly called atheroma. While lipid contents in atheromas are common, some lesions are purely fibrous (Fig. 1). Certain fibrous lesions may, in fact, not be atheromas, but rather responses to injury by

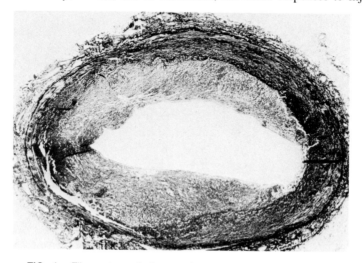

FIG. 1. Fibrous type of atheroma in coronary artery. H & E ×16.

1

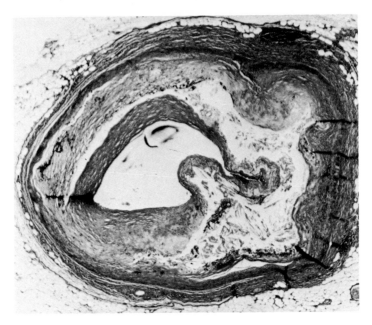

FIG. 2. Coronary artery with one large parite. The lipid content includes cholesterol crystals and shows focal calcification. The fibrous wall covering the lipid is focally thin. H & E, × 12.

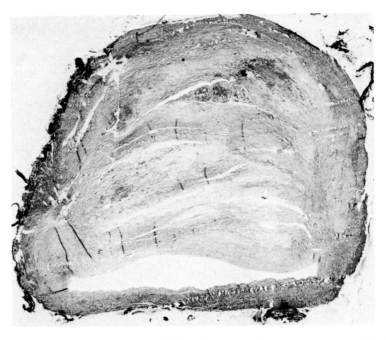

FIG. 3. Coronary artery showing a multiplicity of parites leading to a narrow, eccentric, slitlike lumen. H & E, × 12.

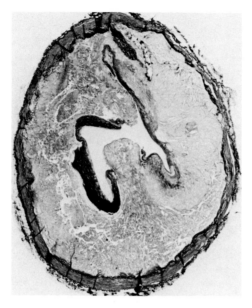

FIG. 4. Coronary artery with circumferential distribution of lipid material. The fibrous layer separating the lipid material from the lumen is thin and has ruptured at two sites. Elastic tissue stain, ×13.

jetlike streams of blood flowing through proximal segments narrowed by atheromas. In some fibrous lesions or in fibrous components of lipid-containing atheromas, there may be lightly staining areas that stain positively for fat. Osborn (2) called the process "collipid" (collagen plus lipid).

The most common type of atheroma results from a highly complex alteration of the intima in which collagen, varying numbers of fat-containing foam cells, and interstitial lipids (with or without crystal formation) participate. A characteristic of lipid accumulation is its association with a fibrous wall on the luminal side of the accumulation (Fig. 2). So strong is the process of fibrous walling of lipid accumulation that Osborn (2) designated the accumulation and its fibrous encasement as one structure, the "parite."

In the minority of segments showing major obstruction of the lumen, only one parite is apparent. Each parite is characterized by an accumulation of amorphous or crystalline lipids walled on the lumen side by fibrous tissue. In most significantly obstructive atheromas, however, a series of parites is more common than one parite (Fig. 3). According to Osborn, the parite is built up by a migration of foam cells from the lumen angles of the atheroma into the substance of the lesion. This would give an episodic character to the progression of atherosclerosis (3).

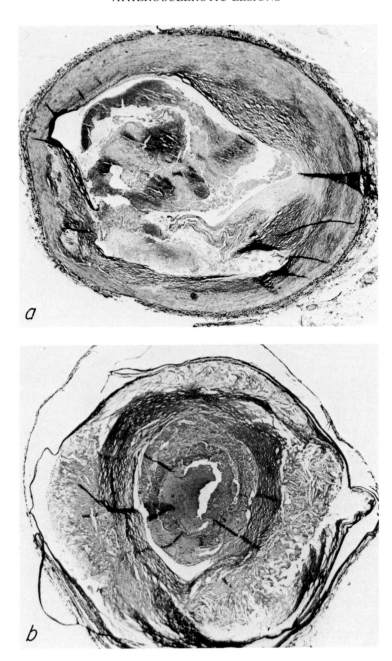

FIG. 5. Thrombosis of atherosclerotic arteries. **a**: Coronary artery. The fibrous covering of a parite has ruptured; the lumen contains a complicating thrombus. Elastic tissue stain, × 15. **b**: Basilar artery. The lumen is occluded by a thrombus. The related fibrous tissue covering the lipid of atheromatous disease has not ruptured. Elastic tissue stain, × 13.

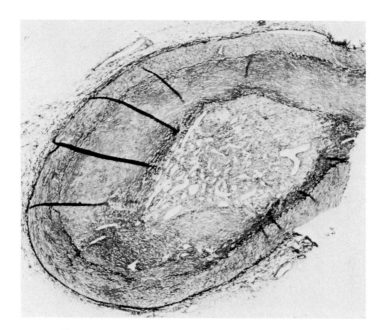

FIG. 6. An organized thrombus in a coronary artery. The original lumen has been narrowed by atherosclerosis and now contains a vascular plexus through which only restricted flow is possible. Elastic tissue stain, × 15.

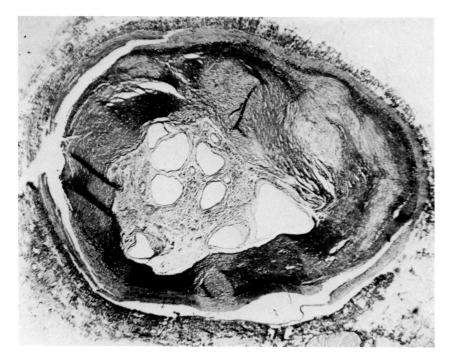

FIG. 7. Coronary artery shows wide channels of a recanalized thrombus through which effective flow had been demonstrated angiographically during life. From Zollikofer et al. (17), with permission.

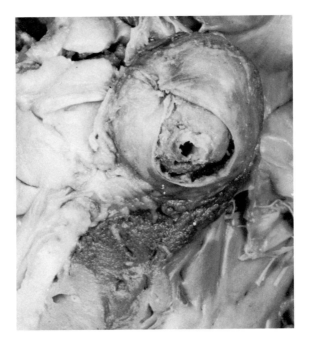

FIG. 8. Specimen of partially opened aneurysm of right coronary artery. The interior of the aneurysm shows a thrombus with a central lumen.

Secondary Changes in and Complications of Atheroma

Calcification

Calcification in atheromas appears to be simply an indication that the involved part of the lesion is old. This process occurs either in accumulations of extracellular lipid or in collagen, the sites of collipid change. Foci of calcification may be seen in those atheromas causing severe stenosis as well as in those with minimal stenosis of the lumen. The latter situation, when observed, is usually seen in the elderly and may mean that the lesion began many years earlier but did not progress (3).

Hemorrhage into Atheromas

Hemorrhage into atheromas, especially into those with a large lipid component, is common. One theory of the origin of hemorrhage is that it is derived from the capillaries that may occur (but are usually not numerous) in atheromas (4–8). The other view is that fragmentation of the fibrous layer of the parite nearest the lumen allows blood from the arterial lumen to extravasate into the lipid accumulation of the atheroma (9–11) (Fig. 4). While hemorrhage into an atheroma entails certain potential consequences, including thrombosis, it does not, of itself, commonly cause significant luminal narrowing.

Thrombosis

Typical thrombosis of a coronary artery usually means underlying atherosclerosis of varying degree, often significant (12–14). Serial sections of thrombosed segments of arteries may show an underlying rupture of the fibrous wall (Fig. 5a) of the related plaque, while in other thrombosed segments, the arterial wall appears not to have been disturbed (15,16) (Fig. 5b).

Thrombi are usually less than 5 mm long. While the lumen is classically occluded, mural thrombi may be seen, leaving some of the lumen intact.

The fate of thrombi may be lysis with either disappearance or organization. Organization of thrombi in atherosclerotic segments is slower than in thrombi present in nonatheromatous vessels. The end product of organization is vascular connective tissue in the original lumen (Fig. 6). While the completely organized thrombus is at times called a "recanalized" thrombus, this term usually is not to be taken to mean restitution of the original lumen. In exceptional cases, the organized thrombus is represented by a small number of wide vessels through which a significant flow of blood may occur (17) (Fig. 7).

Aneurysm

While some atrophy of the arterial media occurs beneath the atheroma, aneurysms do not usually form in vessels other than the abdominal aorta. When an aneurysm results, it usually contains a thrombus—but without occlusion of the lumen (18) (Fig. 8). This thrombus, however, has the potential for fragmentation and embolism (19).

Variation in Luminal Shape in Atheromatous Segments

The principal effect of the atheroma is that it encroaches on the lumen, and the shape of the narrowed lumen depends on the distribution of the atheroma (3). If the atheroma is distributed circumferentially, the lumen lies in a central position and thus may be called a central lumen (Fig. 9a). If the atheroma fails to involve the full circumference of the vessel, the resulting narrowed lumen is called eccentric.

Eccentric lumens are always narrow. Two types are observed: One is slitlike, and the other varies in shape, in some instances being circular. We call an eccentric lumen that is not slitlike polymorphous eccentric (Fig. 9b). In the eccentric slitlike lumen, the length of the slit often nearly approaches the diameter of the original lumen (Fig. 9c). Depending on angiographic projection, the latter process may be one cause of false negative angiograms (20,21). We observed an inordinately high incidence of slitlike lumens among angiographic false negative segments (20).

Vlodaver and I (3) studied histologic sections of 200 coronary arterial segments having significantly obstructive atherosclerosis to determine the relative incidence of the three types of lumens just named (Fig. 10). The distribution was as follows: central lumen, 30.5%; eccentric polymorphous, 40.5%; and eccentric slitlike, 29%. The distribution was essentially the same for each major coronary artery.

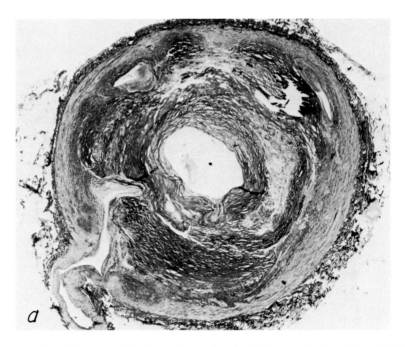

FIG. 9a. Central lumen resulting from atherosclerosis. The lumen of a branch is occluded by the atheroma in the parent vessel. Elastic tissue stain, × 15.

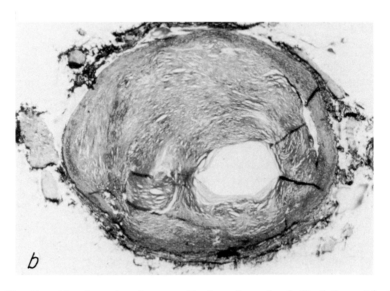

FIG. 9b. Eccentric polymorphous lumen resulting from atherosclerosis. Elastic tissue stain, × 17.

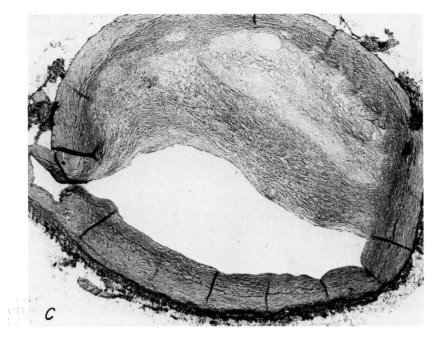

FIG. 9c. Eccentric slitlike lumen resulting from atherosclerosis. The lumen leads to a parent branch. Elastic tissue stain, × 20.

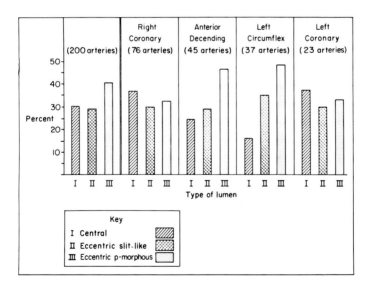

FIG. 10. Distribution of types of lumens in 200 coronary arteries. From Vlodaver and Edwards (3), with permission.

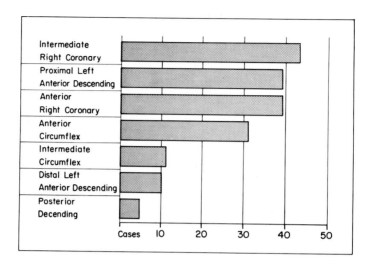

FIG. 11. Incidence of grade 2 or greater atherosclerosis in coronary arteries in each of 50 cases of obstructive coronary atherosclerosis. *Anterior,* proximal segment. *Intermediate segment of right,* segment between marginal and posterior descending. *Intermediate segment of left circumflex* lies distal to origin of marginal branch. From Vlodaver and Edwards (3), with permission.

DISTRIBUTION OF OBSTRUCTIVE LESIONS

To observe the distribution of significant lesions in the coronary system, Vlodaver and I (22) studied 50 hearts from patients with significant coronary atherosclerosis (41 males, 9 females). The most common sites of significantly obstructive coronary atherosclerosis, in order of decreasing frequency, were between the marginal and posterior descending origins of the right artery and the anterior descending and proximal segments of the right and left circumflex arteries (Fig. 11). Our studies (22) found no regular distribution of atheromas in coronary arteries with respect to the surfaces of the heart (Fig. 12).

Regarding the cerebral arterial supply, it is now well known that obstructive atherosclerotic lesions may be present both in the major intracranial and in the cervically located carotid and vertebral arteries.

In surgically accessible segments, the common carotid bifurcation and the adjacent segment of the internal carotid artery are the most common sites of involvement (23–25), followed in decreasing order by the proximal segments of the vertebral arteries and the left subclavian, right subclavian, and innominate arteries. Of the surgically inaccessible segments, the siphon of the internal carotid artery is most commonly affected.

Multiple lesions are frequently seen in patients with cerebrovascular disease, with surgically accessible lesions alone being more common than a distribution of lesions that includes surgically inaccessible segments (25).

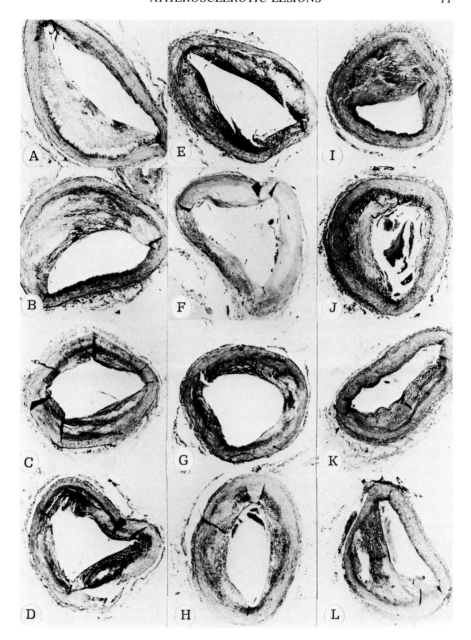

FIG. 12. Sites of atheromas in right coronary artery. Multiple cross sections taken approximately 4 mm apart along the entire course of the right coronary artery from its origin to the origin of the posterior descending. Each segment has the same orientation with respect to the surface of the heart. a, The most proximal segment; l, the most distal segment. The varying orientations of atheromatous plaques with respect to the surface of the heart and the occurrence of uninvolved segments are illustrated. From Vlodaver et al. (22), with permission.

Studying the distribution of obstructive lesions in the arteries of the lower extremity, Haimovici (26) found that multiple lesions were common. The various distributions led to certain groupings, the four most common (in order of decreasing frequency) being (a) tibial arterial only, (b) superficial femoral-popliteal-tibial, (c) popliteal-tibial, and (d) superficial femoral-popliteal-tibial and aortoiliac. The deep femoral artery, significantly, was usually free of disease.

REFERENCES

1. Singer, A. (1963): Segmental distribution of peripheral atherosclerosis. *Arch. Surg.*, 87:384.
2. Osborn, G. R. (1963): *The Incubation Period of Coronary Thrombosis*, p. 190, Butterworths, London.
3. Vlodaver, Z., and Edwards, J. E. (1971): Pathology of coronary atherosclerosis. *Prog. Cardiovasc. Dis.*, 14:256.
4. Paterson, J. C. (1936): Vascularization and hemorrhage of the intima of arteriosclerotic coronary arteries. *Arch. Pathol.*, 22:313.
5. Paterson, J. C. (1938): Capillary rupture with intimal hemorrhage as a causative factor in coronary thrombosis. *Arch. Pathol.*, 25:474.
6. Horn, H., and Finkelstein, L. E. (1940): Arteriosclerosis of the coronary arteries and the mechanism of their occlusion. *Am. Heart J.*, 19:655.
7. Nelson, M. G. (1941): Intimal coronary artery hemorrhage as a factor in the causation of coronary occlusion. *J. Pathol. Bact.*, 53:105.
8. Roberts, J. T. (1945): The role of the small vessels and nerves of the heart in heart failure, coronary artery thrombosis and cardiac pain. *Med. DC*, 14:483.
9. Benson, R. L. (1926): The present status of coronary arterial disease. *Arch. Pathol.*, 2:876.
10. Leary, T. (1935): Pathology of coronary sclerosis. *Am. Heart J.*, 10:328.
11. Clark, E., Graef, I., and Chasis, H. (1936): Thrombosis of the aorta and coronary arteries, with special reference to the "fibrinoid" lesions. *Arch. Pathol.*, 22:183.
12. Spain, D. M., and Bradess, V. A. (1960): The relationship of coronary thrombosis of coronary atherosclerosis and ischemic heart disease. A necropsy study covering a period of 25 years. *Am. J. Med. Sci.*, 240:701.
13. Gould, S. E., and Ionnides, G. (1968): Diseases of the coronary vessels. *Pathology of the Heart*, Third Edition, edited by S. E. Gould, p. 545. Charles C Thomas, Springfield, Illinois.
14. Lawson, M. (1968): Thrombosis in coronary heart disease. *Br. Heart J.*, 30:151.
15. Friedman, M. (1975): The pathogenesis of coronary plaques, thromboses, and hemorrhages: An evaluative review. *Circulation*, 51,52 (*Suppl* III):34.
16. Baba, N., Bashe, W. J., Jr., Keller, M. D., Geer, J. C., and Anthony, J. R. (1975): Pathology of atherosclerotic heart disease in sudden death. I. Organizing thrombosis and acute coronary vessel lesions. *Circulation*, 51,52 (*Suppl.* III):53.
17. Zollikofer, C. L., Vlodaver, Z., Nath, H. P., Castaneda-Zuniga, W., Valdez-Davila, O., Amplatz, K., and Edwards, J. E. (1980): Angiographic findings in recanalization of coronary arterial thrombi. *Radiology*, 134:303.
18. Kalke, B., and Edwards, J. E. (1968): Localized aneurysms of the coronary arteries. *Angiology*, 19:460.
19. Schwartz, C. J., Mitchell, J. R. A., and Hughes, J. T. (1962): Transient recurrent cerebral episodes and aneurysm of carotid sinus. *Br. Med. J.*, 1:770.
20. Vlodaver, Z., Frech, R., Van Tassel, R. A., and Edwards, J. E. (1973): Correlation of the antemortem coronary arteriogram and the postmortem specimen.*Circulation*, 47:162.
21. Arnett, E. N., Isner, J. M., Redwood, D. R., Kent, K. M., Baker, W. P., Ackerstein, H., and Roberts, W. C. (1979): Coronary artery narrowing in coronary heart disease: Comparison of cineangiographic and necropsy findings. *Ann. Int. Med.*, 91:350.
22. Vlodaver, Z., Neufeld, H. N., and Edwards, J. E. (1972): Pathology of coronary disease. *Sem. Roentgenol.*, 7:376.
23. Schwartz, C. J., and Mitchell, J. R. A. (1961): Atheroma of the carotid and vertebral arterial systems. *Br. Med. J.*, 2:1057.
24. Blaisdell, F. W., Hall, A. D., Thomas, A. N., and Ross, S. J. (1965): Cerebrovascular occlusive disease. Experience with panarteriography in 300 consecutive cases. *Calif. Med.*, 103:321.

25. Hass, W. K., Fields, W. S., North, R. R., Kricheff, I. I., Chase, N. E., and Bauer, R. B. (1968): Joint study of extracranial arterial occlusion. II. Arteriography, techniques, sites, and complications. *J. A. M. A.*, 203:961.
26. Haimovici, H. (1967): Patterns of arteriosclerotic lesions of the lower extremity. *Arch. Surg.*, 95:918.

*Noninvasive Techniques for Assessment of
Atherosclerosis in Peripheral, Carotid, and
Coronary Arteries*, edited by Thomas F.
Budinger, et al. Raven Press, New York
1982.

Natural History of Human Atherosclerotic Lesions: Changes in Luminal Configuration

Seymour Glagov* and Christopher K. Zarins**

Departments of Pathology and Surgery**, University of Chicago,
Chicago, Illinois 60637*

NONUNIFORMITY OF LESIONS

Human atherosclerosis is an obliterative and destructive disease of the arterial trunks, the large elastic arteries, and the muscular distributive arteries. It is characterized by focal intimal accumulation of lipids, cells, and matrix elements, which encroach on the lumen. The process may also be accompanied by sclerosis and thinning of the media, with an associated increase in outside vessel diameter. Such dilatations do not necessarily increase the luminal diameter, for an intimal lesion and/or its associated complications may be sufficiently pronounced to result in a net narrowing or obstruction of the lumen.

Although the disease is generally progressive, lesions have shown histologic evidence of healing and organization, implying that they need not progress steadily to lumen obstruction and that changes in their consistency and configuration over time are not necessarily progressive. Lesions may also show sharply demarcated and abutting zones of contrasting organization and composition, suggesting that lesion formation and/or healing may be episodic, that new lesions may form on old lesions, or that adjacent, once discrete lesions may enlarge to collide, coalesce, or overlap one another.

The configuration and functional consequences of an atheromatous deposit depend, in large measure, on the diameter and location of the affected vessel. An atheromatous deposit large enough to nearly obliterate a coronary artery would be of no functional significance in the aorta; moreover, atherosclerosis does not occur or progress at the same rate throughout the arterial tree.

While most individuals with severe aortic disease are likely to have coronary artery involvement as well, mesenteric and renal arteries are usually spared—even in the presence of severe aortic disease. Some individuals with severe aortic disease, nonetheless, have only slight or moderate coronary artery atherosclerosis, while others may have more serious disease in the coronary arteries than in the aorta.

Such findings suggest that the unique hemodynamic conditions in the coronary circulation not only predispose them more to atherogenesis than other arteries of the same size but also determine the relative sparing or involvement of the coronary arteries in comparison to the aorta. The composition of coronary lesions may also be expected to differ from that of lesions in other arteries of similar size. Having appeared earlier, lesions in coronary arteries are likely to be more advanced than those in other vessels; furthermore, having appeared under conditions of greater mechanical stress, lesions in coronary arteries are likely to contain more matrix fibers and more evidence of secondary disruption. The natural history of lesion configuration therefore depends on a series of factors, both general and local, which determine the time of lesion initiation as well as its growth rate, composition, and localization. Lesions should not be considered uniform in structure or composition, even in the same individual or artery.

EVOLUTION OF LESIONS

Observers of human and experimental disease have studied several morphologic types of lesions and reached a number of conclusions about the likely progression from one type to another. Early, focal, intimal lesions contain serum components and often occur preferentially over preexisting diffuse intimal fibrocellular thickenings. Concomitantly, or subsequently, cells accumulate in the intima. These cells are often laden with lipid vacuoles, but much of the intimal lipid remains extracellular. It is not known if the initial intimal swellings are widespread and evanescent and evolve to form focal lesions, due to some additional specific stimulus, or if each swelling already represents a nascent lesion. Injury to endothelial cells has been considered a possible critical event both for stimulation of intimal proliferation by mitogenic factors and for enhancing intimal ingress or increasing serum lipids. Such precursor "microinjuries" are difficult to document in human tissue and would be impossible to appraise on angiography without some marker of altered intimal permeability. The early fatty streak or dot, which contains lipid and lipid-filled cells, also accumulates matrix macromolecules, including glycosaminoglycans and formed fibrils and fibers, such as basal lamina, collagen, and elastin, in close association with the cells.

As intimal lesions increase in volume, two other features become manifest: a decrease in cellularity at the core of the lesion and the formation of a fibrous zone between the lesion and the arterial lumen. The change in the center of the lesion has been interpreted as a form of necrosis, possibly due to isolation of the interior of the lesion from oxygen and metabolites. In any case, the center is often soft, friable, granular, and pultaceous, resembling the gruel from which the term atherosclerosis takes its prefix. The fibrous zone adjacent to the lumen consists of cells and organized connective tissue, largely smooth muscle and collagen. It sequesters the lesion from the lumen, and its surface shape conforms to the generally concave configuration of the vessel interior. It may become as thick as the underlying media or remain a relatively narrow zone, but it is usually uniform in thickness throughout. The typical advanced, uncomplicated plaque is thus an eccentric intimal thickening with a softened, friable center, bracketed on one side by the media and on the lumenal side by a fibrous zone or cap.

Three major complications result in more complex structural formations. Lesions may ulcerate, i.e., become disrupted, so that their deep contents are exposed directly to the lumen. Whether this is a result of mechanical trauma, a defect in the fibrous cap, a change in consistency of the interior, or some sudden change in lesion nutrition is not known. In any event, exposure of the lesion's contents to the bloodstream may lead to either or both of the other complications—thrombogenesis at the lesion surface or entry of blood from the lumen into the plaque interior. Although either of these complications may be expected to increase the effective volume of the plaque, discharge of the lesion contents into the lumen could also diminish plaque volume. Vasa vasorum in and about lesions are another potential source for hemorrhages into plaques, resulting in, or complicating, plaque disruption.

The formation of thrombi on plaques may cause luminal occlusion in arteries of small caliber, such as the coronary arteries, but would not necessarily occlude the aorta unless the disease is very extensive and confluent. Aortic atherosclerotic aneurysm formation is indeed accompanied by encircling thrombus formation. A patent channel within the thrombus, however, usually permits continued flow, and microscopic examinations show sequential organization of layer after layer of thrombus, leaving only a fibrous remnant of the media. The wall of an atherosclerotic abdominal aortic aneurysm is thus composed of atrophic media, atherosclerotic plaque, fibrous tissue layers (which probably represent organized thrombus), and layers of partially organized thrombus. Layered patterns of fibrous tissue deposition, suggesting thrombus organization, can be difficult to distinguish from the intrinsic fibrous component of the plaque. Organized and organizing thrombi, convincingly distinct from underlying plaques, can also be seen in smaller arteries.

At any stage of development of an advanced lesion, calcium deposition may be quite prominent. This may indicate that the lesion has been in place for a long time but does not necessarily provide clues to the functional significance or consistency of the lesion as a whole.

Characterization of lesion morphogenesis according to observations of human lesions does not imply that all or even most early human lesions necessarily evolve to become advanced or complicated. Recent studies of the isoenzyme composition of human lesions suggest that not all fatty streaks are converted into advanced fibrous plaques. We do not know why some advanced lesions ulcerate while others appear to be stable, why some calcify more than others, or why some lead to mural atrophy and dilatation of the vessel, while others are consistent with the preservation of normal outer diameters and a fairly well preserved media. It has not been shown that induced or spontaneous resorption of mobilizable components of advanced lesions will result in predictable changes in lesion size and/or configuration, nor has it been demonstrated that a change in lesion size or configuration in one site indicates a similar or parallel change in a lesion elsewhere.

CONFIGURATION OF LESIONS

Photographs or diagrams of atherosclerosis usually present lesions as bulges or mounds projecting into the lumen of an arterial cross section. Such representations are deceptive, for they are based on specimens fixed by immersion after excision. When vessels are fixed while distended at controlled, approximately normal pressures, their lumens remain nearly circular on cross section—even when marked stenosis by eccentric lesions is present. Viewed in longitudinal planes of section (i.e., parallel to the direction of flow, as on angiograms), lesions appear as irregular luminal narrowings. The luminal surface of a lesion thus generally conforms to the circumferential curvature of the vessel, but the lumen appears tapered on longitudinal projection.

Since lesions are usually eccentric, angiographic visualization by opacification of artery lumens may be deceptive. Viewed in one longitudinal plane, a lesion may appear to have little effect on luminal diameter. Viewed in an orthogonal projection, the same lesion may appear to be quite obstructive. When vessels are viewed end-on, i.e., in the direction of flow, adjacent stenosed and unstenosed segments are likely to be superimposed. As a result, severely obstructive lesions may be masked by lesser lesions.

When viewed en face, lesions in straight portions of arteries tend to appear oval and elongated in the direction of flow, but this effect may be obliterated by early confluence of adjacent lesions. Other lesion outlines and shapes are associated with curves, bends, and branchings. Deposits at branch ostia occur mainly as oval plaques at the ostial inlet opposite the flow divider and as oval or triangular plaques downstream from the flow divider. Plaques do not appear at the edge of the divider except when all lesions show extensive confluence.

Surface Configuration of Early Lesions

The surface configurations of vessels tending to develop focal atheromatous lesions also show a diffuse, concentric form of fibrocellular intimal thickening devoid of the usual focal features of atherosclerotic lesions. This change is not itself obstructive and may occur in dilated vessels whose luminal diameter is greater than normal. Intimal thickening of this type does not appear on angiography and should be difficult to assess by visualizing the lumen. The fatty streak or dot is relatively flat and linear rather than oval. In normally distended vessels, the surfaces of such lesions conform to the curved surface of the adjacent uninvolved intima. Since the lesions are only several cell layers thick, vessel narrowing should be almost imperceptible. Microscopically, the normal endothelial surface is smooth and regular, with only the contours of nuclei projecting from the surface. The surface of an early lesion tends to become bumpy and irregular as cells and fibers accumulate in the intima before the fibrous cap forms. The bumps and crevices, however, are only one to two cells deep, even when the lesions are many more cell layers thick.

When the fibrous cap forms, the overlying endothelium is applied directly to a regular fibrocellular layer oriented circumferentially, with the endothelium at times in close association with a newly formed internal elastic membrane. This transition from a linear or circular fatty streak to a partially encircling eccentric plaque with a necrotic center implies a change in consistency of the lesion. Whether or not this change could be detected as a change in the luminal surface of an artery is not clear. In small vessels, such changes could result in perceptible changes in plaque volume compared with the lumen. In large vessels, however, it is more likely that radiographically demonstrated irregularity or roughness of the intimal surface is due to irregular involvement by adjacent plaques or to complications occurring in some plaques.

Surface Configuration of Advanced Lesions

It will be recalled that the lateral edges of advanced plaques do not generally form elevated or overhanging margins. Lateral plaque edges almost always slope to join the uninvolved adjacent intima in a continuous surface. More prominent edges may be evident at the distal margins of plaques, but a careful study of these features in distended arteries remains to be done. The fibrous cap and adjacent arterial media, over uninvolved or less involved portions of the vessel, thus form a nearly continuous circle on cross section. The irregularities corresponding to advanced plaques on longitudinal projection correspond to the side-by-side arrangements of adjacent plaques along the vessel length. When such plaques collide or coalesce, they may exaggerate demonstrable deformations. It is also conceivable that rough surfaces due to close proximity of individual plaques are smoothed when lesions coalesce.

Complications of advanced lesions also alter their configuration and apparent size. Thrombosis or plaque hemorrhage may appear to be plaque growth, while organization either of plaque thrombi or plaque hemorrhages may appear to be reduction of atherosclerosis. Since these effects might be expected to produce more irregularity of plaque surface than normal plaque growth and organization, determination and recording of the precise sequential positions of reference calcific deposits on complementary projections might help distinguish plaque increase by growth from plaque increase or deformation by complications.

Resorption of plaque constituents under regression regimens, furthermore, could change plaque consistency and, therefore, plaque configuration. This might decrease plaque size, but it might also cause plaques to ulcerate as deformations result from plaque collapse. Such an effect might conceivably be due to differential absorption at the plaque interior rather than the fibrous subintimal layer.

The relationship of plaque morphology and configuration to the appearance of the lumen, as demonstrated by indirect methods, requires more study. It is essential that such postmortem morphologic correlative studies include careful fixation of normally distended vessels.

Noninvasive Techniques for Assessment of
Atherosclerosis in Peripheral, Carotid, and
Coronary Arteries, edited by Thomas F.
Budinger, et al. Raven Press, New York
1982.

Commentary

Gardner C. McMillan

Atherosclerosis, Hypertension, and Lipid Metabolism Section,
Division of Heart and Vascular Diseases, National Heart, Lung, and Blood Institute,
National Institutes of Health, Bethesda, Maryland 20205

You have had a grand tour through arteriosclerosis as it is seen by the pathologist in routine or specially prepared specimens. If I were to characterize what you heard using a single word, it would be "variability."

Variability in what? Variability in the architecture of lesions. No family of disorders is more pleomorphic than arteriosclerosis. Variability also applies to the plasticity of the lesions, that is, their ability to change, whether in terms of progression or regression, composition or the way the lesion evolves.

The word "episodic" can be used to indicate an abrupt change in plasticity after intervals of relative stability. It is a highly variable process and, in the present state of knowledge, largely unpredictable.

I recommend a recent paper by Dr. Michael DeBakey (1), in which he illustrates his experience, on a case-by-case basis, with the progression or failure to progress over time of coronary, carotid, and other lesions as seen by angiography.

There are remarkable differences among individual patients. Dr. DeBakey illustrates lesions that apparently have been stable for as long as 20 years, while in an adjacent part of the same arterial tree, there may have been no change or an accretion of new lesions. In other patients, he has shown that major progressions of lesions have occurred within a year or two. These are phenomena which pathologists cannot grasp using autopsy studies, but they are real enough and are another occurrence included under the term "variability."

Variability in composition: There are fat-rich and fat-poor lesions. You have seen fat very deeply embedded in tissues; you have seen superficial fat. You have seen lesions of cellular and fibrous nature; lesions having calcium; blood in the form of hemorrhage as well as blood elements in the form of thrombi. All such lesions are highly variable in composition.

These phenomena occur in constantly changing vessels. This has not been emphasized commonly in the pathological literature but was emphasized here today. The vessels are plastic; they elongate. One of the characteristic changes a vessel goes through during life is elongation, and tortuous, corkscrew-like vessels will develop when the length of the vessel can no longer be accommodated in a straight line within the organ space. In addition, vessels become ectatic. Distension may develop due to such pathological changes as turbulence, pressures on the vessel walls, and so forth. So we see another aspect of variability. The lesions are discrete, but they are grounded in a vessel and that vessel is changing.

Several months ago, Dr. Blankenhorn raised the question of rate of change. Such cumulative phenomena are not easily detected pathologically, but he proceeded to search the existing literature to determine the severity of atherosclerosis at 5-year intervals of chronological age. (This sequential approach is logically flawed, but it is the best one available.) He came to the conclusion from autopsy data (2) that arteriosclerotic lesions spread over the surface of the aorta (expressed as a percentage of surface) at the rate of about 1.5 percent per year. In terms of femoral lesions according to angiographic data, he determined that arteriosclerosis progresses at the rate of about 2 percent per year. You have to weigh this generalization about rate of change against the earlier remark that there are people who have highly stable lesions. At some period in their lives, they manifest a susceptibility which brings them to clinical attention. They are then said to be at high risk since they do have lesions, yet those lesions may remain remarkably stable.

A variability factor that was not discussed is the question of flux. We have said that lesions have a highly variable composition, that they exhibit change. It is possible to express that thought in terms of flux of elements of plaques, either entering or formed *in situ*, then digested or removed.

It is not a concept that is easy to approach, although it might be a basis for diagnostic techniques. Any approach to it is likely to be flawed, because we do not know whether lesions become areas of excessive flux or are "watersheds" for it. There is evidence in the animal experimental literature for both concepts, and it is clear that a given lesion, according to its composition, may be resistant to changes in terms of flux, whereas another lesion may be highly susceptible.

An implication of what you have read here is that there will also be dynamic consequences, changes in elasticity, changes in the deformability of plaques with each pulse beat. There are well-known changes in pulse rate propagation, and redispersion of energy in the form of turbulence, etc.

The pathology of the lesions implies that they have dynamic consequences, but it tells us very little about them. It is indeed a major hope that the *in vivo* diagnostic techniques may allow them to associate the variability of lesions as seen pathologically with their functional behavior.

REFERENCES

1. DeBakey, M. E. (1976): Patterns of atherosclerosis and rates of progression. In: *Atherosclerosis Reviews Vol. 3*, edited by Paoletti, R. and Gotto, A. M., Jr. Raven Press, New York.
2. Blankenhorn, D. H. (1980): Estimated rates of progression and regression of human femoral and coronary atherosclerosis in 45-year-old men, pp. 715–718. In: *Atherosclerosis V, Proceeding of the Fifth International Symposium*, edited by Gotto, Smith, and Allen. Springer-Verlag, New York.

Noninvasive Techniques for Assessment of Atherosclerosis in Peripheral, Carotid, and Coronary Arteries, edited by Thomas F. Budinger, et al. Raven Press, New York 1982.

Clinical Need for Noninvasive Detection, Quantification, and General Characterization of Lesions in Peripheral Arteries

Robert W. Barnes

Department of Surgery, Medical College of Virginia, Virginia Commonwealth University, Richmond, Virginia 23298

Atherosclerotic peripheral arterial disease may cause abnormal arterial enlargement (aneurysm) or progressive vascular obstruction (stenosis or occlusion, arteriosclerosis obliterans). Aneurysms are often asymptomatic but may be complicated by rupture, thrombosis, or distal embolization of thrombotic or atheromatous debris. Arteriosclerosis obliterans is initially asymptomatic but may eventually cause muscular pain with exercise (claudication), resting ischemic pain, ulceration, or gangrene.

Contrast arteriography remains the diagnostic standard for detection of peripheral arterial disease; however, its expense, discomfort, and risk restrict its indication to candidates for vascular reconstruction. Noninvasive diagnostic techniques, both morphologic (imaging) and physiologic (hemodynamic), may be used in peripheral arterial disease for disease detection, anatomic localization, assessment of functional impairment, prognostic evaluation, perioperative monitoring, and follow-up evaluation.

DISEASE DETECTION

Early detection of asymptomatic disease is particularly important in arterial aneurysm prior to the serious complications of rupture, thrombosis, or embolism. Because aneurysms usually do not alter blood pressure or flow, they are best evaluated by morphologic noninvasive techniques. Aneurysms are usually palpable, but they may be obscured by obesity and mistaken for a tortuous vessel or an overlying soft tissue mass. The lumen of an aneurysm may be of normal caliber as a result of mural thrombus, which limits the diagnostic value of contrast arteriography in such circumstances. Because the risk of rupture of an aneurysm is proportional to its size, the most useful noninvasive techniques are those that can report the overall dimensions of the aneurysm.

Arteriosclerosis obliterans is usually detectable by characteristic clinical symptoms and signs—pulse deficits and arterial bruits. Several conditions may, however, mimic arterial occlusive disease, including neuromuscular (low back) disorders, diabetic neuropathy, and arthritis. Arterial obstruction may coexist with these conditions, furthermore, yet not be the cause of the patient's complaints.

Symptoms of arterial insufficiency are attributable to alterations in blood pressure or flow at rest or following exercise. Physiologic noninvasive techniques have thus been particularly helpful in detecting arterial occlusive disease and discerning true claudication from the "pseudoclaudication" of neurospinal disease, ischemic rest pain from diabetic neuritis, and ischemia from nonischemic ulceration.

ANATOMIC LOCALIZATION

Definition of the regional extent of arterial disease is important in surgical therapy planning. In an abdominal aortic aneurysm, for example, the surgeon should know whether the aneurysm extends proximal to the renal arteries and whether there is associated peripheral or visceral arterial occlusive disease. In arteriosclerosis obliterans of the lower extremities, the distribution of disease is conveniently classified into regions of arterial inflow and outflow (runoff). Inflow vessels include the abdominal aorta and the iliac and common femoral arteries. Outflow arteries are the superficial femoral, popliteal, tibioperoneal, and pedal vessels.

An important surgical precept is the need to reconstruct arterial inflow vessels prior to revascularizing arterial outflow. In patients with multisegmental arterial occlusive disease, an essential diagnostic objective is to define the relative magnitude of disease in the inflow and outflow vessels. Arterial reconstruction of proximal inflow vessels is of more lasting benefit than distal revascularization.

FUNCTIONAL ASSESSMENT

Early arteriosclerosis obliterans may be revealed only by altered blood pressure or flow during periods of circulatory stress, such as exercise or reactive hyperemia following temporary limb ischemia. In the absence of symptoms at rest, limb blood flow may be normal. The presence of arterial obstruction may nevertheless result in circulatory energy losses detectable as abnormal pressure gradients and dampening of the pulsatility of the circulation. The degree of abnormality of these hemodynamic indices, both at rest and during exercise or reactive hyperemia, is a measure of the functional deficit. With progressive arterial obstruction, blood flow may be subnormal at rest, with resultant rest pain or tissue necrosis (ulceration or gangrene).

PROGNOSTIC EVALUATION

An important goal of diagnostic evaluation is the accurate prediction of the natural history or outcome of medical or surgical therapy in peripheral arterial disease. An abdominal aortic aneurysm less than 5.0 cm in diameter, for example, has a likelihood of rupture of less than 15%, whereas an aneurysm of greater than 6.0 cm has a rupture risk exceeding 50%, thus justifying surgical repair of all but the highest-risk patient. Important prognostic objectives of noninvasive diagnostic evaluation of arteriosclerosis obliterans may include prediction of success of proximal (inflow) reconstruction in multisegmental disease, patency of distal bypass procedures, benefit from lumbar sympathectomy for unreconstructable limb ischemia, or healing at a given degree of amputation for severe arterial insufficiency.

PERIOPERATIVE MONITORING

The success and safety of vascular reconstruction are enhanced by objective monitoring before, during, and immediately after operation. Preoperative indices of the presence and relative magnitude of inflow or outflow arterial disease are important in choosing the most appropriate reconstructive procedure. Intraoperative monitoring of the integrity of the revascularized segments and the status of the distal vascular bed can establish the success of the operation and detect those complications (thrombosis, embolism) most readily corrected intraoperatively. Postoperative monitoring can predict the long-term success of the procedure and promptly detect and correct any early postoperative complications.

FOLLOW-UP EVALUATION

Selection of a particular treatment for arterial disease should be based on a sound understanding of the natural history of the disorder and the efficacy of various types of therapy. Many therapeutic approaches are, unfortunately, empirical and not based on objective epidemiologic data. One of the most promising applications of noninvasive diagnostic techniques is in developing objective, quantitative data about the course of vascular disease and the effect of treatment. Small aortic aneurysms may be accurately followed by morphologic studies and their incidence and rates of enlargement defined. Both morphologic and physiologic techniques may be used to identify and follow the course of arteriosclerosis obliterans, which, in most patients, does not require surgical therapy. Such objective indices may enhance epidemiologic assessment of the efficacy of means to control traditional risk factors in order to limit progression or induce regression of peripheral atherosclerosis.

Finally, longitudinal noninvasive studies permit objective evaluation of the integrity of vascular reconstruction and the development of late disease progression or complications. If begun promptly, such studies may help save limb or life.

Noninvasive Techniques for Assessment of
Atherosclerosis in Peripheral, Carotid, and
Coronary Arteries, edited by Thomas F.
Budinger, et al. Raven Press, New York
1982.

Clinical Needs: Carotid Artery Disease

D. E. Strandness, Jr. and Brian L. Thiele

*Department of Surgery, University of Washington School of Medicine,
Seattle, Washington 98195*

The most obvious clinical need in treating atherosclerosis of the carotid arteries is to detect it at a stage when institution of therapy will prevent not only its progression but also its sequelae. This will be attainable only when the following goals have been achieved: (a) accurate identification of those patients at risk; (b) development of methods sensitive enough to detect the disease in its earliest phases; and (c) definition of the stage in the disease at which progression can be halted, and—hopefully—regression can be effected by institution of therapy.

Accurate, noninvasive testing procedures may offer significant benefit in several clinical situations in terms of both planning management and avoiding the complications common to arteriography.

It is generally accepted that patients with symptomatic cerebral ischemia should undergo arteriography. There are, however, patients in this category without disease of the extracranial arteries who might be spared arteriography if the absence of disease in their neck vessels could be accurately documented. At the opposite end of the spectrum, patients may have symptoms secondary to occlusion of the internal carotid artery, a condition that generally precludes operative intervention and the need for arteriography. Accurate screening to verify internal carotid occlusion would also obviate the need for the invasive studies. While only 5 to 10% of the patient population have normal extracranial arteries or total occlusion, this is a significant number given the magnitude of the overall problem of symptomatic cerebral ischemia.

The second important group of patients are those with asymptomatic neck bruits. The decision to proceed with arteriography is prompted by the knowledge that the presence of a bruit, in and of itself, does not pinpoint its source or the degree of stenosis. Furthermore, despite considerable controversy, there is a large body of opinion that patients with high-grade stenoses should undergo arteriography and possible operation. The direct and some of the indirect tests are capable of detecting such lesions, thus permitting arteriography for a wider range of patients.

An asymptomatic bruit in a patient facing a major operation complicates planning for the procedure. Although (again) controversial, increasing efforts are being made to identify patients with flow-reducing lesions prior to operation, so that correction can be made either prior to, or simultaneous with the anticipated major procedure. One group for which this is urgently needed includes those about to undergo cardiac surgery, during which perfusion pressure may fall to low levels while controlled by the heart-lung machine. Noninvasive screening of these patients may identify those at risk for stroke during or following the operative procedure.

The value of arteriosclerosis therapy has largely been predicated on its relief of symptoms. While this criterion is commonly employed in clinical research, it does have limitations. It would be better not only to cite relief of symptoms as an endpoint, but also to follow objectively morphological changes in the arterial segment in question. This might be accomplished by repetitive angiography, but that approach is simply not feasible with current methods. Imaging techniques, however, do hold considerable promise in this setting, particularly when combined with estimation of the flow changes that can be made at regular intervals during follow-up.

Finally, we present a supposition that at the moment would appear to be heretical: is there a need for arteriography even when operation is contemplated? Does angiography change the operative approach to patients with transient ischemic attacks? In most instances, except for the presence of a total occlusion, the arteriogram does not determine the type of procedure, since this is dictated by the findings of the operation. The reason usually given for arteriography is the need for a complete study of not only the extracranial but the intracranial circulation as well. Disease of the carotid siphon, for example, has been given as a reason for not approaching the carotid bifurcation directly. Mere angiographic demonstration of two lesions in series obviously cannot indicate which of the stenoses is responsible for the patient's symptoms. While demonstration of a second lesion does alert the physician to its presence, the choices of therapy, therefore, must still be largely based on the clinical picture and a qualitative interpretation of the arteriogram. Noninvasive tests can, of course, be of assistance, particularly if the extent and nature of the carotid lesion can be accurately assessed.

The future of this field appears promising—if the noninvasive tests become sensitive enough and if they give answers to some of the still open questions. Development of the appropriate technology will have to be accomplished by well planned, carefully controlled clinical trials.

Noninvasive Techniques for Assessment of Atherosclerosis in Peripheral, Carotid, and Coronary Arteries, edited by Thomas F. Budinger, et al. Raven Press, New York 1982.

Noninvasive Technology and Carotid Artery Disease: An Overview[1]

James F. Toole

Department of Neurology, Bowman Gray School of Medicine, Wake Forest University, Winston-Salem, North Carolina 27103

Each year, nearly 600,000 people in the United States become stroke victims, most as the direct result of atherosclerosis. Approximately 40% of these die within a month, and at least two-thirds of those who survive have permanent disability. The population of the United States currently includes 2½ million disabled survivors of stroke.

With the aging of our population and the control of heart disease and cancer, the problem of stroke will take on increasing importance for health care and economic planners. Behavioral abnormalities secondary to cerebrovascular disease, including post-stroke dementia, personality changes, mood and memory impairment, and loss of specific skills, will also increase and must be addressed.

It is estimated that about 70% of strokes are caused by atherosclerosis. Carotid artery disease is responsible for nearly half of all infarctions due to atherosclerosis and accounts for about 20% of all strokes. Over 90% of carotid plaques lie in the neck of patients with infarction due to carotid disease; about half experience a transient ischemic attack (TIA) within a month prior to infarction. Regarding the two main possibilities, occlusion or embolism, as many as 60% of patients with carotid disease may have their stroke secondary to embolism from a carotid plaque. This group is likely to have warning TIAs.

The variety of definitions and methods used to collect and analyze data on TIAs has made it extremely difficult to get reliable information. The incidence rate for TIAs approaches 5/1,000/year in the population aged 65 and over—between 4 and 10 times that of the controlled population for stroke—and may even reach 35% within a 4-year period. TIA is thus one of the best indicators for impending cerebral infarction. About 30% of patients with TIAs of the carotid artery have other clinically

---

[1]Author's note: Some material contained herein is excerpted from the report of the cerebrovascular disease panel of the Working Group on Arteriosclerosis, National Heart, Lung, and Blood Institute, January, 1979.

29

detectable signs of arteriosclerosis in the carotid arteries, such as murmur or abnormalities in the collateral circulation through the external carotid artery.

From the therapeutic viewpoint, carotid, coronary, and intracranial arteriosclerosis must be considered together, because:

1. Many (though not all) of the risk factors are the same for each.

2. Arteriosclerosis in all these sites is very similar, and histopathological, cytopathological, and biochemical features of the lesion are the same, with very minor variations.

3. Complicated lesions (thrombosis, stenosis, ectasia, plaque ulceration, and plaque hemorrhage) occur in all these sites, and even though their clinical expression depends on the vascular bed involved, their pathological process is the same in each.

4. Two-thirds of patients with intra- and extracranial arteriosclerosis succumb to myocardial infarction.

5. Postmortem examinations of Americans have shown that carotid and coronary artery arteriosclerosis become evident in the second decade of life and have a parallel evolution. This raises the possibility that examining the accessible extracranial carotid artery can give important clues to the state of coronary circulation.

Because the carotid bifurcation may be the most easily sampled segment of the arterial system, it is vital to develop methods to ascertain safely, reliably, and inexpensively the presence of asymptomatic lesions in this system in order to ascertain the presence of disease in less accessible arteries.

Most stroke care is delivered in smaller hospitals; research and development programs are thus needed to design a system requiring minimal technical expertise to apply new devices accurately and to facilitate diagnostic interpretation. This must include unbiased testing in centers not involved in the original research and development, with appropriate studies to assess the sensitivity, specificity, reliability, and cost benefit to the health care system of new equipment.

Technical development must be encouraged by facilitation, not restriction, of inventiveness and innovation, and technology transfer should include support of demonstration centers and workshops training biomedical scientists and clinical investigators. We addressed this need when we assessed the reliability of continuous-wave (CW) Doppler ultrasound for predicting arteriographic findings of stenosis or occlusion at the carotid bifurcation. We compared the results of ultrasound testing and cervical carotid arteriography in 195 arteries of 105 patients with suspected carotid artery disease. We found that the Doppler method provided no significant predictive value in arteries classified as up to 50% stenosed. In stenoses greater than 50%, but not occluded, CW ultrasound predicted the angiogram results with 70% reliability. The greatest correlation between the two methods was obtained in those arteries identified by the Doppler evaluation as being 75 to 95% stenosed.

These results indicate that much useful information can be obtained from Doppler evaluation but that the poor correlation between it and the arteriogram leaves much to be desired. The importance of a positive study must be stressed, because noninvasive evaluation can identify individuals with stenosis exceeding 50% with a reliability exceeding bedside examination and is therefore an important supplement for patient evaluation.

THE NEED FOR CLINICAL TRIALS

Twenty-five years ago, patients with cerebrovascular diseases were usually classified as having had a "stroke" or "cerebrovascular accident." No further subclassification of the disorder was considered necessary because, as a rule, the management of all was the same—bed rest and supportive care. With the advent of medical and surgical therapy for treating cerebrovascular insufficiency, it became necessary to diagnose patients accurately during the premonitory stages. This led to pathoanatomic classification of cerebrovascular disease, precise identification of the transient ischemic attack syndrome and its pathogenesis, identification of extracranial atherosclerotic cerebrovascular syndrome, and most recently, extracranial and intracranial bypass operations. A plethora of diagnostic techniques and therapies has been developed to identify and remove arterial sources for cerebral emboli, each with a basis in logic, but few affording sufficient numbers of patients for objective analysis of their utility.

The inability to draw firm conclusions from such studies goes hand in hand with their lack of proper methodologic control. The following deficiencies have been noted in most studies:

1. Imprecise diagnostic criteria; poor angiographic/CCT and anatomic correlation.

2. Lack of proper sampling techniques.

3. Retrospective rather than prospective analysis of data.

4. Poor coordination of multi-institutional studies.

5. Too few cases for statistical analysis.

6. Rapidly evolving technology, which renders systems obsolete before they can be evaluated.

7. Observer bias, which leads to enthusiastic claims and premature marketing of new symptomatic and diagnostic systems.

8. Effects of the profit motive.

To assess the effectiveness of diagnostic techniques, one must know first the natural history of the disorder. Biostatistical methods are usually required for this, and as a consequence, clinical trials or randomized studies have proliferated. Public concerns about research ethics, federal interest in quality control, and physicians' interests in the legal aspects of such quality assessment have increased concern about adverse implications of randomized trials. To be valid, the data accumulated must be amenable to statistical analysis; a clinical trial worth doing is worth doing properly. Biostatistical input must thus be planned in order to design appropriate sample sizes and make discrete hypotheses. Prospective studies are therefore a cost-effective method for evaluating new technologies when manufacturers or clinicians cannot afford to make their own assessment.

THE PATIENT WITH AN ASYMPTOMATIC BRUIT

A unique category of asymptomatic patients has atherosclerosis evidenced by a bruit in the neck. Detection of such bruits by auscultation is a recently developed skill; the technique for auscultation of the arteries in the neck needs to be better defined, and medical students and physicians need to be better instructed in it. This technique, which can be taught to allied health professionals, has the potential for identifying patients at particularly high risk and should perhaps be incorporated into mass screening programs for the detection of hypertension. How best to manage these patients is still a matter of some dispute, but all agree that careful follow-up of this high-risk population is justifiable.

A survey to identify asymptomatic carotid bruits in 1,746 people over 45 years of age in Evans County, Georgia, revealed them in 2.7% of men and 5.8% of women, with 5.1% in blacks and 4.1% in whites. Follow-up for an average of 6 years saw major stroke in 10.3% of the population with bruits but in only 3.9% of those without bruits. Surprisingly enough, the side of the body affected by stroke was opposite the side with bruit in one-half of the cases. Mortality from stroke and myocardial infarction was 12.7% in those with bruits but only 6.2% in those without; bruit is thus a predictor for stroke and myocardial infarction.

A controversial aspect of stroke prevention is the advisability of arteriography and operation for patients with asymptomatic carotid bruits, which indicate atherosclerotic plaques at the carotid bifurcation. Studies have demonstrated that the asymptomatic carotid bruit reflects an increased risk of cerebral infarction, which can be significantly reduced by carotid endarterectomy—if the accompanying complications of surgery can be controlled.

We need to know how best to determine the significance of a carotid bruit, because not all are indicative of atherosclerosis. Means for characterization exist but need further development. A battery of noninvasive tests seem to be the best answer so far.

RECOMMENDATIONS

1. The public and physicians must be made aware of the significance of transient ischemic attacks. Health care providers must understand the emergent nature of TIAs and be prepared to act when they occur.

2. Epidemiologic methods must be applied to identify individuals at increased risk of stroke.

3. Because 8.7% of strokes occur during hospitalization, special attention must be given to this group.

4. Atherosclerosis in its early phases must be reliably detected and characterized, so that preventive measures can be initiated.

5. A screening and referral mechanism for the stroke-prone individual is needed, such as an improved system for noninvasive imaging of the arteries supplying the cerebral circulation.

6. Noninvasive techniques are not sufficiently refined to indicate degrees of severity and types of atherosclerosis in the carotid arteries of the neck. A well-designed study to determine the degree of correlation between noninvasive imaging and the postmortem appearance of the carotid lesions is necessary.

7. Clear identification of the possible relationship between severity of lesions in one site (carotid, coronary, or intracranial) as a predictor of lesions in another site is necessary, and the means for imaging them simultaneously or in sequence must be developed.

8. Because of the high postoperative mortality following coronary bypass surgery or carotid endarterectomy, the feasibility of a combined surgical approach to carotid and coronary disease should be determined.

BIBLIOGRAPHY

1. Borhani, N., and Greenhouse, A. (1972): Joint Council/Community Program Task Force Recommendations for Medical Education and Community Program Priorities. *American Heart Association.*
2. Canadian Cooperative Study Group (1978): A randomized trial of aspirin and sulfinpyrazone in threatened stroke. *N. Engl. J. Med.,* 299:53.
3. Collaborative Group for the Study of Stroke in Young Women (1975): Oral contraceptives and stroke in young women: Associated risk factors. *J.A.M.A.,* 231:718.
4. Garraway, W. M., Whisnant, J. P., Furlan, A. J., Phillips, L. H., Kurland, L. T., and O'Fallon, W M. (1979): The declining incidence of stroke. *N. Engl. J. Med.,* 300:449.
5. Genton, E., Barnett, H. J. M., Fields, W. S., Gent, M., and Hoak, J. C., (Study Group on Antithrombotic Therapy) (1977): Cerebral ischemia: The role of thrombosis and antithrombotic therapy. *Stroke,* 8:150.
6. Goldstein, M., Bolis, L., Fieschi, C., Gorini, S., and Millikan, C. H. (1979): *Cerebrovascular Disorders and Stroke, Vol. 25: Advances in Neurology.* Raven Press, New York.
7. Haerer, A. F., Gotshall, R. A., Conneally, P. M., et al. (1977): Cooperative study of hospital frequency and character of transient ischemic attacks. III. Variations in treatment. *J.A.M.A.,* 238:142.
8. Jonas, S., Klein, I., and Dimant, J. (1977): Importance of Holter monitoring in patients with periodic cerebral symptoms. *Ann. Neurol.,* 1:470.
9. Kannel, W. B., Dawber, T. R., Sorlie, P., and Wolf, P. A. (1976): Components of blood pressure and risk of atherothrombotic brain infarction: The Framingham study. *Stroke,* 7:327.
10. Kartchner, M. M., and McRae, L. P. (1977): Noninvasive evaluation and management of the "asymptomatic" carotid bruit. *Surgery,* 82:840.
11. Machleder, H. I., and Barker, W. F. (1977): Noninvasive methods for evaluation of extracranial cerebrovascular disease: A comparison. *Arch. Surg.,* 112:944.
12. Mitchell, J. R. A., and Schwartz, C. J. (1962): Relationship between arterial disease in different sites: A study of the aorta and coronary, carotid and iliac arteries. *Br. Med. J.,* 1:1293.
13. Pessin, M. S., Duncan, G. W., Mohr, J. P., Poskanzer, D. C. (1977): Clinical and angiographic features of carotid transient ischemic attacks. *N. Engl. J. Med.,* 296:358.
14. Popp, A. J., and Chater, N.: Extracranial-to-intracranial vascular anastomosis for occlusive cerebrovascular disease: Experience in 110 patients. *Surgery,* 82:648.
15. Sahs, A. L., Hartman, E. C., and Aranson, E. M. (1976): Guidelines for stroke care. U.S. DHEW, Public Health Service, Washington, D.C.
16. Schwartz, C. J., and Mitchell, J. R. A. (1961): Atheroma of the carotid and vertebral arterial systems. *Br. Med. J.,* 2:1057.
17. Siekert, R. G. (1976): *Cerebrovascular Survey Report for Joint Council Subcommittee on Cerebrovascular Disease (revised).* Whiting Press, Rochester, Minnesota.
18. Solberg, L. A., McGarry, P. A., Moossy, J., Tejada, C., Loken, A. C., Robertson, W. B., and Donoso, S. (1968): Distribution of cerebral atherosclerosis by geographic location, race and sex. *Lab. Invest.,* 18(5):144.

19. Soltero, I., Liu, K., Cooper, R., Stamler, J., Garside, D. (1978): Trends in mortality from cerebrovascular diseases in the United States, 1960–1975. *Stroke*, 9(6):549.
20. Strong, J. P., Correa, P., and Solberg, L. A. (1968): Water hardness and atherosclerosis. *Lab. Invest.*, 18:(5):160.
21. Tower, D. B. (1979): *National Research Strategy for Neurological and Communicative Disorders*, NINCDS, U.S. DHEW, NIH.

Noninvasive Techniques for Assessment of
Atherosclerosis in Peripheral, Carotid, and
Coronary Arteries, edited by Thomas F.
Budinger, et al. Raven Press, New York
1982.

Clinical Need for Noninvasive Assessment of Atherosclerotic Lesions in Coronary Arteries

Harold T. Dodge

*Department of Medicine, Division of Cardiology, University of Washington,
Seattle, Washington 98105*

Although the death rate from the cardiovascular diseases has been decreasing since 1960, they accounted for approximately 47% of disease-related deaths in 1976 (1). Of these, coronary heart disease has the highest mortality and morbidity; in 1976, it caused 65% of deaths due to cardiovascular disease.

To reduce or prevent the mortality, morbidity, and high cost of coronary heart disease, we need more effective methods of early detection and quantification of lesions and of determining their clinical course. Only then can therapeutic measures for favorably influencing the course of coronary atherosclerosis be developed and evaluated.

The most widely used method for the detection of coronary atherosclerosis is the exercise stress test, in which ST-segment changes induced by stress indicate ischemic heart disease. However, false positive and false negative results of such testing are frequent (2–6). Furthermore, this test does not measure the *extent* of coronary artery disease. In most studies, myocardial imaging during exercise and rest using thallium 201 has been more sensitive than exercise testing for detecting coronary stenoses $\geq$ 75% of vessel diameter (7–9). For myocardial imaging combined with conventional stress testing, the rate of detection of such stenoses is reported to be 89% or greater (7,9). Thallium 201 imaging during coronary vasodilatation induced by dipyridamole has given results similar to those from imaging during exercise stress (10). However, thallium 201 screening gave false negative results in approximately 20 to 40% of patients with significant coronary lesions (11) and, accordingly, is of limited value in screening of asymptomatic patients and in quantitative assessment of the extent of coronary disease. Furthermore, atherosclerotic lesions producing $\leq$ 50% stenosis cannot be detected by thallium imaging. Studies in experimental animals indicate that with improved myocardial imaging techniques, these methods can be made more sensitive, and coronary artery stenoses of $\geq$ 40% may be identified (12). Coronary stenoses of 47% have been detected in dogs using nitrogen 13 ammonia and positron emission-computed tomography (13).

Assessment of global and regional left ventricular performance by radionuclide angiography at rest and during exercise has a reported sensitivity of 95% for detection of coronary stenoses of $\geq$ 50% (14). However, the method cannot detect all diseased arteries, does not provide quantifying information, and probably will not detect $\leq$ 50% narrowing of the arteries.

In collaboration with Dr. B. G. Brown and his associates in Los Angeles, my colleagues and I (15) have been assessing a computer-assisted technique, developed by Brown and co-workers in my laboratory, for measuring coronary arteries and their stenotic lesions using coronary arteriograms. This technique is apparently accurate within 150 microns in measuring arteries within 4% of the actual percentage of stenosis. The results of some using this technique show that it could meet the need for evaluating noninvasive methods of assessing coronary atherosclerosis in man. In one such study (16), computer-produced coronary lesion measurements were compared with visual estimates of severity by five experienced angiographers. As reported in earlier studies, the visual estimates varied considerably. This variability was particularly marked in assessment of 50 to 70% stenoses, where the average standard deviation was 12.9%, compared with 2.9% for the computerized method. The angiographers also tended to overestimate the severity of lesions. This study points out the dangers of using visual estimates of lesion severity, as seen in coronary arteriograms, as a standard for evaluating other methods. Such visual estimates have been the standard of comparison in most studies evaluating myocardial imaging and radionuclide cineangiography as noninvasive detectors of significant coronary disease. Clearly, a more accurate standard is required.

The dimensions of apparently normal as well as stenotic segments of coronary arteries will change in response to drugs and reflexes. Nitroglycerin dilates the coronary arteries of subjects with and without coronary artery disease (17,18). Nitroglycerin and nitroprusside will also dilate approximately 80% of stenotic coronary artery segments (19), and verapamil has a similar effect on stenotic segments (20). Propranolol often causes constriction, and strength of hand grip is associated with degree of constriction (B. G. Brown, *personal communication*). To assess and quantify such changes accurately, the absolute dimensions of the apparently normal segments and stenotic segments of the coronary arteries must be determined, since the degree of change varies among segments, and since expressing the change as percentage of narrowing may thus give misleading results. Furthermore, knowledge of the absolute dimensions of the stenosis allows one to determine its physiologic effect by measuring changes in the extent of stenosis as resistance and arterial pressure drop across the lesion (15). Clinicians would be greatly aided by indirect techniques sensitive enough to detect these changes.

Noninvasive techniques for measuring the severity of coronary disease would be of considerable clinical value. Physiologic studies in experimental animals (21) have shown (and it is generally accepted for man) that lesions causing less than 40 to 50% coronary arterial stenosis do not significantly interfere with coronary blood flow, even during stress. Only when lesions produce greater than 85 to 90% stenosis do they interfere with resting flow (21). Unstable angina and subendocardial infarction, two common clinical syndromes, are reported to have coronary artery stenotic segments with minimum diameters of 0.88 ± 0.14 mm (92%) and 0.654 $\pm$ 0.08 mm (95%), respectively (22). Here again, the actual length and diameter of the lesions are preferable to percentage of narrowing, because they allow computation of the effects of the stenoses on resistance and pressure drop across the lesions (22).

Perhaps the most important applications of techniques for more accurately quantifying coronary artery disease will be to determine the rate of progression of lesions and the effects of various therapeutic interventions on that rate or on regression of lesions. Coronary angiography has been and is being used for such studies. Gensini and co-workers (23), using visual estimates of severity, found disease progression in 76% of unoperated patients with coronary disease over an average follow-up period of 26 months. In studies of 88 lesions in 25 patients (24), Raffenbeul and co-workers found that over an average interval of 1 year, approximately 79% of the lesions were unchanged, 16% progressed, and 5% regressed. In our collaborative studies with Dr. Brown, we analyzed 225 lesions by computer in 21 patients (over 10 lesions per subject) electively catheterized 18 months after the initial study. Approximately 20% of the lesions had progressed, 10% had improved, and the remainder were unchanged (25). Lesions of all stages progressed, not just the severe ones. Because these data were obtained in an ongoing, randomized, blind study of platelet-inhibiting drugs, they cannot be considered as defining the natural history of coronary artery lesions. However, it is clear that at this rate of progression, an intervention providing 50% benefit in the rate of progression could be evaluated using only 44 patients (472 lesions). This information points out the need and the potential application for good, quantitative noninvasive techniques to evaluate the severity of coronary disease and also for future studies to evaluate the effect of interventions on the course of coronary atherosclerosis. To date, such studies as the Multiple Risk Factor Intervention Trial have relied on the occurrence of clinical events, making them very large, expensive, epidemiologic studies, difficult to conduct. Furthermore, studies of lesions may make it possible to determine which stenotic lesions remain unchanged, which progress, and why. It is of interest that in each of the previously cited studies, regression of lesions was observed with a frequency that varied from 2.4 to 10% (23–25), yet the nature of such regression of atherosclerosis is little understood.

It does seem clear that better noninvasive techniques to detect and quantify coronary atherosclerosis would have important clinical and research applications. These applications would very likely include studies to better determine the natural history of coronary disease and the influence of abnormalities such as hyperlipemia on the rate of progression and the development of more effective methods of evaluating therapies for preventing progression or causing regression of lesions. Clinical applications might well include the serial measurement of coronary vascular lesions to assess the effectiveness of therapy in individual patients. These applications await the development of reliable noninvasive techniques that have been carefully evaluated to determine their sensitivity, specificity, and reproducibility. Controlled trials might be necessary for such evaluations. Methods for quantifying coronary arterial lesions using cineangiograms of the coronary arteries will also prove important in evaluating new noninvasive methods.

REFERENCES

1. Fifth Report of the Director of the National Heart, Lung and Blood Institute. DHEW Publication No. (NIH) 78-1415, February 28, 1978, p. 32.
2. Redwood, D. R., Borer, J. S., and Epstein, S. E. (1976): Whither the ST segment during exercise? *Circulation*, 54;703.
3. Bruce, R. A., and McDonough, J. R. (1969): Stress testing in screening for cardiovascular disease. *Bull. NY Acad. Med.*, 45:1288.
4. Froelicker, V. F., Thomas, M., Pillow, C., and Lancaster, M. D. (1974): An epidemiologic study of asymptomatic men screened with exercise testing for coronary heart disease. *Am. J. Cardiol.*, 34:770.
5. Paine, T. D., Dye, L. E., Roitman, D. I., Sheffield, L. T., Rackley, C. E., Russell, R. O., and Rogers, W. J. (1978): Relation of graded exercise test findings after myocardial infarction to extent of coronary artery disease and left ventricular dysfunction. *Am. J. Cardiol.*, 42:716.
6. Epstein, S. E. (1978): Value and limitations of the electrocardiographic response to exercise in the assessment of patients with coronary artery disease. *Am. J. Cardiol.*, 42:667.
7. Ritchie, J. L., Trobaugh, G. B., Hamilton, G. W., Gould, K. L., Narahara, K. A., Murray, J. A., and Williams, D. L. (1977): Myocardial imaging with thallium-201 at rest and during exercise. Comparison with coronary arteriography and stress electrocardiography. *Circulation*, 56:66.
8. Bailey, K. I., Griffith, L. S. C., Rouleau, J., Strauss, H. W., and Pitt, B. (1977): Thallium-201 myocardial perfusion imaging at rest and during exercise. Comparative sensitivity to electrocardiography in coronary artery disease. *Circulation*, 55:78.
9. Bodenheimer, M. M., Banka, V. S., Fooshee, C. M., and Helfant, R. H. (1979): Comparative sensitivity of the exercise electrocardiogram, thallium imaging and stress radionuclide angiography to detect the presence and severity of coronary heart disease. *Circulation*, 60:1270.
10. Albro, P. C., Gould, K. L., Wescott, R. J., Hamilton, G. W., Ritchie, J. L., and Williams, D. L. (1978): Non-invasive assessment of coronary stenosis by myocardial imaging during pharmacologic coronary vasodilatation. *Am. J. Cardiol.*, 42:751.
11. Ritchie, J. L., Zaret, B. L., Strauss, H. W., Pitt, B., Berman, D. S., Shelbert, H. R., Ashburn, W. L., Berger, H. J., and Hamilton, G. W. (1978): Myocardial imaging with thallium-201: A multicenter study in patients with angina pectoris or acute myocardial infarction. *Am. J. Cardiol.*, 42:345.
12. Gould, K. L. (1978): Assessment of coronary stenoses with myocardial perfusion imaging during pharmacologic coronary vasodilatation. *Am. J. Cardiol.*, 42:761.
13. Gould, K. L., Schebert, H. R., Phelps, M. E., and Hoffman, E. J. (1979): Non-invasive assessment of coronary stenosis with myocardial perfusion imaging during pharmacologic coronary dilatation. V. Detection of 47 percent diameter stenosis with intravenous nitrogen-13 ammonia and emission-computed tomography in intact dogs. *Am. J. Cardiol.*, 43:200.
14. Borer, J. S., Kent, K. M., Bacharach, S. L., Green, M. V., Rosing, D. R., Seides, S. F., Epstein, S. E., and Johnston, G. S. (1979): Sensitivity, specificity and predictive accuracy of radionuclide cineangiography during exercise in patients with coronary heart disease. *Circulation*, 50:572.
15. Brown, B. G., Bolson, E., Frimer, M., and Dodge, H. T. (1977): Quantitative coronary arteriography. Estimation of dimensions, hemodynamic resistance and atheroma mass of coronary artery lesions using the arteriogram and digital computation. *Circulation*, 55:329.
16. Koh, D., Mitten, S., Stewart, D. K., Bolson, E., and Dodge, H. T. (1979): Comparison between computerized quantitative coronary angiography and clinical interpretation. *Circulation II*, 59,60:160 *(abstract)*.
17. Gensini, G. G., Kelly, A. E., Dacosta, B. C. B., and Huntington, P. P. (1971): Quantitative angiography: The measurement of coronary vasomobility in the intact animal and man. *Chest*, 60:522.
18. Feldman, R. L., Pepine, C. J., Curry, R. C., Jr., and Conti, C. R. (1979): Different responses to nitroglycerine in large and small coronary arteries. *Circulation II*, 59,60:263.

19. Doerner, T. C., Brown, B. G., Bolson, E., Frimer, M., and Dodge, H. T. (1979): Vasodilator effects of nitroglycerin and nitroprusside in coronary arteries. *Am. J. Cardiol.*, 43:416.
20. Chew, C. Y. C., Brown, B. G., Wong, M., Shah, P. M., Singh, B. N., Bolson, E., and Dodge, H. T. (1980): The effects of verapamil on coronary artery hemodynamics and vasomobility in patients with coronary artery disease. American College of Cardiology, 29th Annual Scientific Session *(abstract)*.
21. Gould, K. L., Lipscomb, K., and Hamilton, G. W. (1974): Physiologic basis for assessing critical coronary stenosis. Instantaneous flow response and regional distribution during coronary hyperemia as measures of coronary reserve. *Am. J. Cardiol.*, 33:87.
22. McMahon, M. M., Brown, B. G., Cukingnan, R., Rolett, E. L., Bolson, E., Frimer, M., Dodge, H. T. (1979): Quantitative coronary arteriography: Measurement of "critical" stenosis in patients with unstable angina and single vessel disease without collaterals. *Circulation*, 60:106.
23. Gensini, G. G., Esente, P., and Kelly, A. (1974): Natural history of coronary disease in patients with and without coronary bypass graft surgery. *Circulation II*, 49,50:98.
24. Raffenbeul, W., Smith, L. R., Rogers, W. J., Mantle, J. A., Rackley, C. E., and Russell, R. O., Jr.(1979): Quantitative coronary arteriography. Coronary anatomy of patients with unstable angina pectoris reexamined one year after optimal medical therapy. *Am. J. Cardiol.*, 43:699.
25. Brown, B. G., Pierce, C. D., Peterson, R. B., Bolson, E., and Dodge, H. T. (1979): A new approach to clinical investigation of progressive coronary atherosclerosis. *Circulation II* 59,60:66

Noninvasive Techniques for Assessment of Atherosclerosis in Peripheral, Carotid, and Coronary Arteries, edited by Thomas F. Budinger, et al. Raven Press, New York 1982.

What the Epidemiologist and Clinical Interventionist Expect and Need for Studies of Atherosclerotic Disease

William R. Harlan and J. Richard Landis

Department of Postgraduate Medicine, Health Professions Education, University of Michigan, Ann Arbor, Michigan 48109

Noninvasive methodology for the study of arterial lesions could radically transform the nature and cost of epidemiological studies and intervention trials. From the perspective of the epidemiologist, it might be well to outline the promise of this methodology and clarify needs and expectations for further methodological development.

Visualization and imaging of the arterial system could open the black box that heretofore has admitted only glimpses (usually one-time views) of the events occurring within the arterial tree (Fig. 1). The impact of following intraarterial events and changes, albeit "through a glass darkly," cannot be overemphasized, because it will disclose many important facts about the natural history of disease and its alteration with therapy.

Currently, large numbers of individuals must be followed, usually prospectively and serially, to determine the relationships between initial characteristics and subsequent development of disease. For example, approximately 6,000 persons were

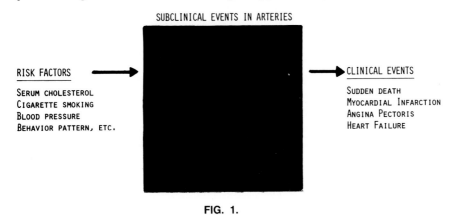

FIG. 1.

followed over three biennial examinations in Framingham, Massachusetts, to discover significant relationships between the initial characteristics and the subsequent development of clinical disease. The requirement for large numbers followed over relatively long periods in this study derives from several characteristics of atherosclerotic disease and from the epidemiologic approach.

First, there is a relatively long latency between initial development of arterial lesions and the clinical events that form the endpoint. Second, the measurement of these endpoints uses means that are relatively insensitive and require frequent assessment. Moreover, the variability in the measurement of these clinical manifestations is considerable. Much of this variability is attributable to different intraarterial biologic events (plaque accretion, thrombosis, etc.) that have the same manifestations. The result is an epidemiologic requirement for large numbers of individuals followed over relatively long periods. The cost is high, but the yields have also been great.

When therapeutic interventions are tested, the problems become more complex, and the size and cost of studies increase. For example, the Multiple Risk Factor Intervention Trial has enrolled more than 12,000 participants in a 6-year study to determine whether or not intervention on the conventional risk factors (cigarette smoking, high blood pressure, and elevated serum cholesterol) will decrease the clinical manifestations of disease. The question is important, and there is no other feasible approach, but, not unexpectedly, this is an expensive undertaking.

How could noninvasive methods change these epidemiologic and intervention studies? The ability to image and measure intraarterial lesions could potentially decrease the interval required to measure changes in arterial lesions, because it would not be necessary to wait for clinical events (Fig. 2). In a corollary manner, the number of subjects required for study might be significantly decreased, and one or two collaborating institutions might provide an adequate number of subjects rather than the 10 to 12 institutions plus a coordinating center that are required by the current strategy. The study efficiency and cost-saving might be changed by a factor of 4 or 5.

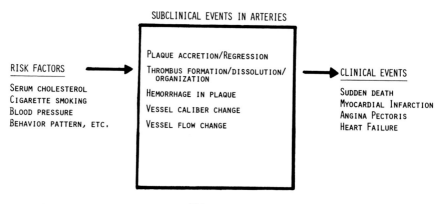

SUBCLINICAL EVENTS IN ARTERIES

RISK FACTORS ➡️

SERUM CHOLESTEROL
CIGARETTE SMOKING
BLOOD PRESSURE
BEHAVIOR PATTERN, ETC.

PLAQUE ACCRETION/REGRESSION
THROMBUS FORMATION/DISSOLUTION/
ORGANIZATION
HEMORRHAGE IN PLAQUE
VESSEL CALIBER CHANGE
VESSEL FLOW CHANGE

➡️ CLINICAL EVENTS

SUDDEN DEATH
MYOCARDIAL INFARCTION
ANGINA PECTORIS
HEART FAILURE

FIG. 2.

Additional information might be provided regarding the association between a risk factor and a specific intraarterial event. For example, it may be possible to determine whether cigarette smoking is related to the propagation of plaque formation or to other events, such as arterial caliber, flow, or thrombosis. Intervention on a specific risk factor might disclose what aspect of the obstructive lesion (plaque, thrombosis, vessel caliber, etc.) was changed by therapy, and whether combinations of interventions are additive or synergistic in affecting luminal obstruction. Additionally, the ability to make serial measurements with little risk to the patient should broaden the degree of atherosclerotic disease that might be studied and extend the age ranges of populations under study.

At present, most prospective epidemiologic and intervention studies are directed toward populations thought to have relatively extensive disease and likely to manifest a clinical event within a reasonable follow-up interval (3 to 5 years). Without a reasonably high likelihood of a clinical event, the number of subjects or the interval of follow-up necessary to gain statistical significance is increased considerably. Therefore, the epidemiology of arterial disease in the younger individual has not been studied but is extremely important in intervention.

What demands would the epidemiologist place on this methodology in order to achieve these important gains in information and cost efficiency? To answer this question, it is important to consider the critical facets of study design for the epidemiologist and interventionist. In study design, the critical variables are: number of subjects, length of observation (which may be combined person-years of study), the extent of change (or δ), and the variability of the measurement and of the biologic change. The ability or power of the study to detect significant changes depends on these variables (1).

For the epidemiologist concerned with the "natural" changes in arterial lesions or the investigator mounting an intervention trial to evaluate therapies, the only study design variable under direct control has been the number of person-years of observation. The extent of change, or δ, is usually the dependent variable. The variability entailed in using clinical manifestations as measurements of change has been well known and accepted, because no other approach was available.

However, the advent of noninvasive methodology potentially capable of improving the accuracy of the change measurement and refining the detection of change alters the situation. The potential for direct measurement of arterial disease is amply demonstrated by many studies (2,3), recently those of Blankenhorn et al. (4,5). But this great promise has an important quid pro quo for the investigator. Improved efficiency in study design can be determined only when the variability is known. An example will illustrate the importance of determining variability before planning a study or trial.

Assume that we wish to plan a study that will disclose the natural history of carotid artery lesions and subsequently explore the efficacy of a therapeutic intervention. Among the decisions to be made by the study planners are the number and type of subjects to be recruited. To carry this example forward, we have made some simplifying assumptions. These include the following:

1. Only clinically significant and potentially reversible arterial lesions will be studied, ranging in degree of obstruction from 40 to 80%.

2. The rate of progressive obstruction/regression is unknown but is in the range of 1 to 20%/year.

3. The variability, which includes the biologic variability *and* the measurement variability, is unknown. We have selected standard deviations of 5, 10, 15, and 20% as reasonable ranges of variability. In the table, these are presented as variances—the squares of the above numbers.

4. Follow-up periods of 1, 2, and 3 years would represent likely periods of observation.

5. The rates of progression are linear over time for the model developed here. However, similar models could be developed, so long as the rate of change can be described as a mathematical function.

6. Statistical significance will be assessed using a one-tailed, paired t-test at the $\rho = 0.05$ level. To ensure that the power of the test is 0.95, the error was also set at $\rho = 0.05$.

The sample size computations for a study of progression are given in Table 1. The contingencies of size of initial lesion (μ_0), time of follow-up (τ), and extent of change (δ) are outlined, assuming that the correlation between initial and subsequent measurement (ρ) is 0.8 and the variance is 25 (or a variability of 5%). Otherwise, for the other combinations of correlation and variance shown in Table 2, the required sample sizes can be obtained directly from Table 1 by multiplying the given sample size by the corresponding factor from Table 2.

For example, if the mean arterial obstruction on entering the study is 50% and the rate of change is 2%/year, significant differences could be detected in as few as 27 subjects in a 2-year period *if* the variance was 25 (σ^2) and the correlation between measurements (ρ) was 0.8. However, if the variance was 225, the required sample size would increase to 243. In practical terms, a study that might be accomplished by one investigator would become a study requiring several centers to recruit subjects and would have to deal with the problems of coordinating all aspects of the study. The multiplier effect on costs would probably be great as well.

Another facet of methodologic needs is illustrated by this example. The natural history of arterial obstruction is an important feature that heretofore has been obscure. For example, it is not certain that the course of atherogenesis is relentlessly progressive or proceeds in a linear manner. It is possible that lesions may progress, remain unchanged, or regress without specific therapy and that these trends may occur in a "stuttering," or rapid-slow, fashion rather than linearly. All of these possibilities, as well as the possibility that lesions may progress in one region while remaining stable or regressing in other areas, would have to be considered in study design. Clearly, long-term observations of this biologic variability have a high priority for study.

The reason for presenting this model is to illustrate the important role that variability plays in design of studies of arteriosclerotic disease. This aspect deserves

TABLE 1. *Required sample sizes for detecting one-tailed increments for $\rho = 0.8$ and $\sigma = 5$*

μ_0	τ	1	2	5	10	20
				δ		
40	1	676.6	169.1	27.1	6.8	1.7
	2	169.1	42.3	6.4	1.5	*
	3	75.2	18.8	2.7	*	*
50	1	433.0	108.2	17.3	4.3	1.1
	2	108.2	27.1	4.2	1.0	*
	3	48.1	11.3	1.7	*	*
60	1	300.7	75.2	12.0	3.0	*
	2	75.2	18.8	2.8	*	*
	3	33.4	7.8	1.2	*	*
70	1	220.9	55.2	8.8	2.2	*
	2	55.2	13.8	2.1	*	*
	3	24.5	5.9	*	*	*
80	1	169.1	42.3	6.8	1.7	*
	2	42.3	10.6	1.6	*	*
	3	18.8	4.5	*	*	*

*$N < 1.0$.
δ = percent change per time period, τ.
μ_0 = size of initial lesion, percent obstruction.
ρ = correlation between initial and successive measurements.

TABLE 2. *Multiplication factors for sample sizes in Table 1 under alternative correlation and variance parameters*

	25	100	225	400
		σ^2		
0.6	2	8	18	32
0.8	1	4	9	16

σ^2 = variance.

exploration by those developing noninvasive technology. Definition of this variability and means of minimizing it should have a high priority when technical development is stabilized and biologic applications are developed. Although the instrumentation is still evolving, it is not too soon to begin this assessment, and this can serve as another means of comparing different technologies and protocols. We do not mean to minimize the importance of validity studies or determinations of sensitivity and specificity, but rather to highlight the importance of variability in epidemiologic studies and intervention trials.

At the risk of appearing pedantic, we would like to outline the sources of variability to afford a road map for those who are persuaded that definition is an important endeavor. The sources of variability are outlined in Table 3. These may be separated into two general categories of variability, measurement and biologic. There is no need to review extensively the sources of measurement variability except to note the important role that the observer/interpreter may play. Many current technologies require that the interpreter determine which point of the arterial obstruction will be measured as maximum and which segment of the artery is "normal", thereby forming the basis for comparison. This has been responsible for considerable variability in arteriographic studies of coronary and femoral lesions (2–5) and will undoubtedly pose problems for noninvasive techniques.

Commonly, our concern about the technologic variability overshadows another important, although less alterable, source of variability-biologic variation. Because we have not had a means of viewing the dynamics of intraarterial events, many investigators have assumed that the process of atherogenesis is a gradual, progressive process that proceeds in a linear manner. Repeat angiographic studies, although relatively few in number, suggest that this view is simplistic and that, in fact, progression and regression occur even without therapy. Moreover, the obstructing lesion apparently may change abruptly in extent and nature and, over a long period, follow a stuttering course of rapid progression, followed by a plateau of change. Clearly, an important priority must be assigned to further assessment of this biologic variability, both short-term (i.e., weeks or months) and long-term (i.e., years).

Rather than laying out an agenda for evaluation of this technology preparatory to designing natural history and intervention trials, we would prefer to stress the importance of these efforts and their critical impact on epidemiologic and intervention studies. If one examines the history of "quantitative" femoral and coronary angiography and of echocardiography, the lessons are clear. Efforts at assessing and minimizing measurement variability were undertaken only after expensive, frustrating, and often unsuccessful attempts had been made to use these methods to evaluate interventions. The more appropriate and less expensive sequence requires evaluation of methodology first. Noninvasive technology has a tremendous potential in clinical investigation, but this potential will not be fully realized without attention to the problems of measurement and biologic variability.

TABLE 3. *Variability in measuring biological changes*

Measurement variability
Instrument
Operator
Observer/interpreter
Biologic variability
Short-term
Long-term

REFERENCES

1. Cohen, J. (1977): *Statistical Power Analyses for the Behavioral Sciences*. Academic Press, New York.
2. Brown, B. G., Bolson, E., Frimer, M., et al. (1977): Quantitative coronary arteriography. Estimation of dimensions, hemodynamic resistance, and atheroma mass of coronary artery lesions using the arteriogram and digital computation. *Circulation*, 55:329.
3. Detre, K. M., Wright, E., Murphy, M. L., et al. (1975): Observer agreement in evaluating coronary angiograms. *Circulation*, 52:979.
4. Barndt, R., Jr., Blankenhorn, D. H., Crawford, D. W., et al. (1977): Regression and progression of early femoral atherosclerosis in treated hyperlipidemic patients. *Ann. Int. Med.*, 86:139.
5. Blankenhorn, D. H., Brooks, S. H., Selzer, R. H., et. al. (1978): The rate of atherosclerosis change during treatment of hyperlipoproteinemia. *Circulation*, 57:355.

Noninvasive Techniques for Assessment of Atherosclerosis in Peripheral, Carotid, and Coronary Arteries, edited by Thomas F. Budinger, et al. Raven Press, New York 1982.

Use of B-Mode Ultrasonic Imaging in the Detection and Evaluation of Experimentally Induced Atherosclerosis in Animals

Sheldon A. Schaffer, Andrew S. Katocs, Jr., and Theresa M. Sapp

Department of Biology, Medical Research Division, American Cyanamid Company, Pearl River, New York 10965

B-mode ultrasonic imaging has great potential for the early detection of arteriosclerotic disease. Like contrast arteriography, ultrasonic imaging can determine the presence and magnitude of arterial lesions. However, unlike arteriography, ultrasonic imaging pictures the arterial wall itself and thus has potential for discriminating among various types of arterial lesions. The ability to describe atherosclerotic lesions as they occur *in situ* and to follow the natural course of their development (or regression) would be invaluable in furthering our understanding of this important disease. Such knowledge would also be of great help in the clinical evaluation of new drugs or other therapies designed to treat this disease.

In scanning human carotid arteries, we (1) and others (2,3) have observed that the ultrasonic images of atherosclerotic lesions vary considerably in character from intensely bright reflections of the ultrasonic signal to nearly sonolucent ones. To investigate the relationships between these different types of ultrasonic images and actual tissue composition, we are studying the ultrasonic image characteristics of lesions induced in animals and obtaining detailed data on actual arterial pathology. This chapter describes our early investigations of ultrasonic imaging in the New Zealand rabbit and the macaque monkey.

Our ultrasonic imaging system was a prototype developed at the Science and Technology Research Center of the New York Institute of Technology. It operates with a transducer frequency of 6 to 11 MHz, and scanning is accomplished mechanically at a rate of 30 Hz. Its depth of focus is variable using interchangeable lenses. For scanning rabbit aortae, we used a 2.5 cm focal length lens and a 1.25 cm lens for scanning monkey carotids. The scanner has a resolution capability of 0.5 mm in range and 0.7 mm in azimuth.

We first used our system to study aortic atherosclerosis induced in male rabbits. (Rabbits are well suited to atherosclerosis studies, since lesions can be induced in them within a relatively short time.) Scanning from the ventral surface, the aorta of the rabbit may be imaged from a region just proximal to the celiac bifurcation to the aortoiliac bifurcation. The scan was made parallel to the long axis of the aorta for an image of a longitudinal slice and perpendicular to this axis for a cross-sectional image. In the normocholesterolemic rabbit, ultrasonic imaging of the aorta showed a clear lumen and smooth, well-defined arterial walls. The average luminal diameter ranged from 6 cm in the lower thoracic aorta to 4 cm in the lower abdominal segment.

We induced atherosclerotic lesions in 20 rabbits by supplementing their diets with either 2% crystalline cholesterol or 2% cholesterol plus 6% peanut oil for periods of from 1 to 6 months. Within the first month, few changes in the aorta were observed. The aortic walls remained smooth and distinct. At 6 to 8 weeks, bright ultrasonic reflections at the arterial wall protrusion into the lumen were observed in many of the animals. These changes were most commonly seen in the ventral wall of the aorta, both in longitudinal and in cross-sectional images. Several of the animals were sacrificed at this point.

The animals were scanned just before sacrifice, and using a reference point on the transducer, the locations of any unusual imaging reflections were marked on the animals' skin. After sacrifice, the mark was aligned with the aorta *in situ* to identify the suspect region. In all cases, unusual ultrasonic reflections accurately indicated an atherosclerotic lesion in the marked aortic segment. These lesions were mostly fatty streaks, microscopically composed of a large amount of lipid, including numerous foam cells. Intimal cell proliferation and accumulation of fibrous connective tissue were also apparent. These lesions were not uniform in thickness, but at their thickest point the intimal lesions were approximately 0.2 mm with an intima:media ratio of 1.

Six animals were examined from 3 to 6 months after the initiation of the high cholesterol diet. In these animals, the frequency of lesions in the ultrasonic images increased. However, the severity of the lesions as measured by brightness or thickness of the reflected ultrasonic signal did not change. These lesions were similar to those induced in the shorter-term cholesterol-fed rabbits, except that intimal thickness increased to about 0.5 mm.

The lesions induced in the cholesterol-fed rabbits were similar in many respects to human fatty streaks, but they did not mimic the more advanced lesions found in man. Even in rabbits fed cholesterol for relatively long periods of time, moreover, the aortic lesions remained diffuse and fairly flat. Therefore, we investigated other animal models of atherosclerosis.

Nonhuman primates, particularly macaques, have been made to develop atherosclerotic lesions demonstrating many features of advanced human disease (4,5). In our preliminary investigations, we found that at least three arterial beds could be imaged in the cynomolgus monkey (Macaca fascicularis) using the ultrasonic scanner—the aorta, the carotid artery, and the femoral artery. The carotid artery was most easily imaged, because for the most part it lies in a single plane parallel to the skin surface.

We undertook a study of the use of B-mode imaging in detecting and analyzing carotid artery atherosclerosis in the cynomolgus monkey, using 15 adult male animals weighing between 4 and 6 kg each. In 10 of the monkeys (group A), atherosclerosis was induced by feeding them a diet containing 2% cholesterol and 10% butter. The remaining five animals (group B) were fed a normal chow diet. All were examined by ultrasonic scanner prior to the experiment and again 3 and 6 months later.

For ultrasonic imaging, the anesthetized animals were placed in a supine position. The neck was carefully shaved to remove all hair. With the probe placed approximately midway between an anterior and lateral position on the neck, the carotid artery could be imaged from just above the clavicle to the carotid bulb. In approximately 70% of the carotid scans, the carotid bulb could be seen clearly, both in longitudinal and in cross-sectional approaches. In the remaining 30%, the carotid bifurcation was positioned behind the mandible and thus could not be imaged with the relatively large ultrasonic probe. Tracking the artery in the longitudinal scans was sometimes difficult, but pulsation of the vessel indicated that the structure seen on the video monitor was an artery.

The luminal diameter of the carotid arteries in these animals ranged from 1.5 to 2.3 mm. The images showed a clear lumen and smooth, distinct walls. No evidence of spontaneous disease was found in any of the animals prior to feeding the cholesterol-rich diets.

Due to technical difficulties, the ultrasonic images observed in 3-month scans were unsuitable for analysis. No data were recorded, therefore, on the presence of carotid artery lesions after the first 12 weeks of the experiment. After 6 months on the cholesterol-rich diet, no bright focal reflections similar to those seen in the aorta of the cholesterol-fed rabbit were seen in group A monkeys; moreover, no changes in luminal diameter were detected. In several images, however, we saw a broadening of the reflections from the arterial walls and an increase in roughness of their luminal surfaces. The magnitude of these changes did not permit any quantitative evaluation of lesion severity, and our failure to obtain satisfactory images of the carotid arteries in all animals precluded the rank ordering of atherosclerotic lesion involvement in group A monkeys. No changes were seen in the carotid artery images of group B animals.

All of the animals were sacrificed at 6 months, and the carotid arteries were removed and examined for gross or microscopic evidence of atherosclerosis. The unstained carotid arteries in group A animals showed grossly a widely varying pattern of disease, and the mean involvement was 53%. In three monkeys, however, the common carotid artery was nearly devoid of lesions, and in four other animals, the incidence of lesions was only 20 to 30%.

Inasmuch as the range of atherosclerosis involvement was of greatest interest in this study, we concentrated our analysis on those arteries showing abundant lesions and those vessels nearly devoid of disease. In two animals, the lesion incidence approached 100%. These lesions were best described grossly as fatty streaks and fatty plaques. Microscopically, they were characterized by moderate intimal thickening (intima:media ratio between 0.5 and 1.25 mm), with numerous intimal foam cells and accumulation of fibrous connective tissue. There was also a striking accumulation of monocytic cells in the intima and the underlying media. In group B animals and in three group A animals, there was neither gross nor microscopic evidence of atherosclerosis.

As mentioned above, the most striking difference between the ultrasonic images of the carotid arteries in the animals with abundant atherosclerotic lesions and those with normal arteries was an apparent thickening of the arterial walls and an increase in roughness of their luminal surfaces. The small caliper of the carotid artery and the relative flatness of the induced lesions made them impossible to measure. Such measurement would require more pronounced lesions. In fact, using our current instrument, with its resolving power of 0.5 mm, intimal lesions more than twice as thick as those seen in this study would be needed before they could be measured with any degree of confidence. A 6-month feeding experiment using the cynomolgus monkey is clearly not long enough to produce lesions of this magnitude.

These preliminary investigations have shown that B-mode ultrasonic imaging can detect early atherosclerotic lesions. The fatty streaks induced in the rabbit were clearly seen. The mild fibrofatty plaques seen in the monkey carotid artery were, however, more difficult to detect. It is evident that longer-term experiments, producing more pronounced arterial lesions, are needed to identify the possible relationships between ultrasonic images of atherosclerotic lesions and their actual pathology.

REFERENCES

1. Hobson, R. W., Berry, S. M., Katocs, A. S., O'Donnell, J. A., Zafar, J., and Savitsky, J. P. (1980): Comparison of pulsed Doppler and real-time B-mode echo arteriography for noninvasive imaging of the extracranial carotid arteries. *Surgery*, 87:286.
2. Green, P. S., Taenzer, J. C., Ramsey, S. D., Holzemer, J. F., Suarez, J. R., Marich, K. W., Evans, T. C., Sandok, B. A., and Greenleaf, J. F. (1977): A real-time ultrasonic imaging system for carotid arteriography. *Ultrasound Med. Bio.*, 3:129.
3. Cooperberg, P. L., Robertson, W. D., Fry, P., and Sweeney, V. (1979): High resolution real-time ultrasound of the carotid bifurcation. *J. Clin. Ultrasound*, 7:13.
4. Kramsch, D. M., and Hollander, W. (1968): Occlusive atherosclerotic disease of the coronary arteries in the monkey (Macaca irus) induced by diet. *Exp. Mol. Pathol.*, 9:1.
5. Armstrong, M. L., and Megan, M. B. (1975): Arterial fibrous proteins in cynomolgus monkeys after progression and regression diets. *Circ. Res.*, 36:256.

Noninvasive Techniques for Assessment of Atherosclerosis in Peripheral, Carotid, and Coronary Arteries, edited by Thomas F. Budinger, et al. Raven Press, New York 1982.

Review of Nonimaging Methods

Robert W. Barnes

Department of Surgery, Medical College of Virginia, Virginia Commonwealth University, Richmond, Virginia 23298

Nonimaging diagnostic techniques in vascular disease may be considered physiologic or hemodynamic because of their sensitivity to alterations in blood pressure or flow. This chapter will briefly review the currently practical instrumentation, techniques, and applications of physiologic diagnostic methods in peripheral arterial and cerebrovascular disease (1).

INSTRUMENTATION

Doppler Ultrasound

The Doppler ultrasonic velocity detector is the most versatile and least expensive device to evaluate peripheral arterial (2), cerebrovascular (3), and venous disease (4). Continuous-wave instruments operating at 5 to 10 MHz may be portable and nondirectional and have audio outputs, or they may be tabletop models with a direction-sensing capability for analogue recording or sound spectral analysis. Doppler instruments may be used for blood velocity analysis and blood pressure measurements in addition to imaging.

Plethysmography

Plethysmographs measure changes in dimension of a portion of the body with each heart beat or with interruption of venous return (venous occlusion plethysmography). Several types of transducers are available, including water [ocular plethysmography (OPG-Kartchner/McRae) (5)], air [pulse volume recorder (PVR) (6), phleborrheograph (PRG) (7), ocular pneumoplethysmograph (OPG-Gee) (8) and (OPG-Zira)], strain gauge (SPG) (9), impedance (IPG) (10), and photoelectric (PPG) (11) methods. Plethysmographs permit pulse waveform analysis (contour, amplitude, timing) and measurement of blood pressure and blood flow [venous occlusion plethysmography (12)].

Phonoangiography

Vascular bruits associated with arterial stenosis may be graphically recorded as an amplitude-time plot (5) or as a spectral display of frequency versus amplitude

(13). Such phonoangiographic techniques are best used to detect and quantify carotid artery bruits.

Isotopes

In addition to radionuclide angiography, isotopes may be used to detect regional blood flow by such methods as xenon-133 washout (14) and arteriovenous shunting by distribution of intraarterially injected radioisotope microspheres (15). Active venous thrombosis may be detected by abnormal uptake of 125-labeled fibrinogen (16).

Electromagnetic Flowmetry

Although most electromagnetic flowmeters are designed to be applied directly to exposed vessels, a noninvasive technique has been designed to assess limb blood flow (17). Although the technique involves sophisticated computerized signal averaging, the method is sensitive only to the pulsatile component of arterial blood flow.

Thermography

The thermograph is a sensitive detector of infrared radiation from the body (18). The method has been used to detect areas of abnormal coolness of the forehead associated with carotid occlusion as well as limb coolness (in peripheral arterial disease) or warmth (in venous disease). The technique is rather expensive and less accurate than many other noninvasive methods.

TECHNIQUES AND APPLICATIONS

Vascular disease may be qualitatively or quantitatively evaluated by measurement of alterations in blood pressure, blood flow, pulse volume, or arterial wall vibrations (bruits).

Blood Pressure Measurement

Whereas resting blood flow is reduced only in advanced arterial occlusive disease, alterations in systolic blood pressure occur fairly early in the clinical course of arteriosclerosis obliterans. The ankle/arm pressure index (API)—ankle systolic blood pressure relative to that of the arm—is the simplest quantitative method of screening for peripheral arterial occlusive disease (19). One's API is normally ≥ 1.0, but in the presence of leg arterial obstruction, the API will be less than 1.0 in an amount proportional to the degree of circulatory impairment. Patients with claudication have an API between 0.5 and 0.9, and individuals with rest pain or gangrene usually have an API < 0.5, with an absolute ankle pressure often less than 50 mm Hg. Localization of arterial obstruction may be assessed by measuring segmental limb blood pressures at the proximal thigh, above-knee, below-knee, and ankle levels using specially designed cuffs (20). These pressures are most readily measured by Doppler ultrasound but may also be determined by plethysmography (21). The latter technique is particularly useful in determining digit blood pressures using strain gauge, photoelectric, or air transducers.

To quantify the function capacity of the circulation to respond to stress, the ankle pressure response to exercise (22) or reactive hyperemia (23) may be determined.

Pressure measurements to screen for carotid occlusive disease may be made using ophthalmodynamometry (ODM) (24) or OPG-Gee (8).

Blood Flow Measurement

Qualitative assessment of altered blood flow velocity may be most simply performed using Doppler ultrasound. The Doppler probe may be positioned along the course of the major arteries to detect alterations in the audio output of the instrument (2). The normally multiphasic arterial signal may be abnormally high-pitched at a stenosis and be monophasic distal to an arterial obstruction. Analogue recording of the velocity signal permits hard-copy recording for qualitative and quantitative assessment of peripheral arterial (25) and cerebrovascular diseases (26). The most sensitive detection of early atherosclerotic stenosis is obtained by sound spectral analysis of the Doppler frequency shifts (27). This technique may become an integral part of Doppler imaging systems in screening for early carotid occlusive disease. It has already been used to determine the pulsatility index in screening for peripheral arterial occlusive disease (28).

Blood flow measurement is feasible using venous occlusion plethysmography (12) and xenon-133 washout determinations (14). However, these techniques are somewhat technically demanding and are more suitable for research. Blood flow measurement in arterial disease is most sensitive when carried out during or after exercise or reactive hyperemia, since resting blood flow may be normal in all but the most advanced stages of arterial disease.

Pulse Waveform Analysis

Pulse waveforms recorded by plethysmography may be analyzed for alterations in pulse contour, amplitude, or arrival time. Segmental limb pulse contour and amplitude alterations are the methods by which the PVR evaluates peripheral vascular disease (6). Attenuation of supraorbital PPG pulse amplitude by compression of the external carotid artery branches may indicate carotid occlusive disease (29). Delay of ocular pulse arrival time is the clue for detection of carotid disease using the OPG-Kartchner/McRae (5) and OPG-Zira methods. Delay of the digit pulse reappearance following temporary limb ischemia is a sensitive index of peripheral arterial occlusive disease (25).

Bruit Assessment

There are two methods of analyzing a vascular bruit. Qualitative recording of the bruit is achieved with the carotid phonoangiograph (5), which depicts an amplitude-time plot on oscilloscope for subsequent storage on a Polaroid photograph. Quantitative assessment of the severity of arterial stenosis is possible by spectral analysis of the frequency content of the bruit (13).

REFERENCES

1. Barnes, R. W. (1979): Noninvasive diagnostic techniques in peripheral vascular disease. *Am. Heart. J.*, 97:241.
2. Barnes, R. W., and Wilson, M. R. (1976): *Doppler Ultrasonic Evaluation of Peripheral Arterial Disease: A Programmed Audiovisual Instruction*, p. 296. University of Iowa Press, Iowa City.
3. Barnes, R. W., and Wilson, M. R. (1975): *Doppler Ultrasonic Evaluation of Cerebrovascular Disease: A Programmed Audiovisual Instruction*, p. 196. University of Iowa Press, Iowa City.
4. Barnes, R. W., Russell, H. E., and Wilson, M. R. (1975): Doppler *Ultrasonic Evaluation of Venous Disease: A Programmed Audiovisual Instruction, 2nd ed.*, p. 220. University of Iowa Press, Iowa City.
5. Kartchner, M. D., McRae, L. P., and Morrison, F. D. (1973): Noninvasive detection and evaluation of carotid occlusive disease. *Arch. Surg.*, 106:528.
6. Darling, R. C., Raines, V. K., Brener, B. V., and Austen, W. G. (1972): Quantitative segmental pulse volume recorder: A clinical tool. *Surgery*, 72:873.
7. Cranley, J. J., Canos, A. J., Sull, W. J., and Grass, A. M. (1975): Phleborrheographic technique for diagnosing deep venous thrombosis of the lower extremities. *Surg. Gynecol. Obstet.*, 141:331.
8. Gee, W., Oller, D. W., and Wylie, E. J. (1976): Noninvasive diagnosis of carotid occlusion by ocular pneumoplethysmography. *Stroke*, 7:18.
9. Whitney, R. J. (1949): The measurement of changes in human limb volume by means of a mercury-in-rubber strain gauge. *J. Physiol.*, 109:5P.
10. Wheeler, H. B., Pearson, D., O'Connell, D., and Mullick, S. C. (1972): Impedance phlebography. *Arch. Surg.*, 104:164.
11. Hertzman, A. B. (1938): The blood supply of various skin areas as estimated by the photoelectric plethysmograph. *Am. J. Physiol.*, 124:328.
12. Brodie, T. E., and Russell, A. E. (1905): On the determination of the rate of blood flow through an organ. *J. Physiol.*, 32:47P.
13. Duncan, G. W., Gruber, J. O., Dewey, C. F., Jr., Myers, G. S., and Lees, R. S. (1975): Evaluation of carotid stenosis by phonoangiography. *N. Engl. J. Med.*, 293:1124.
14. Lassen, N. A. (1964): Muscle blood flow in normal man and in patients with intermittent claudication evaluated by simultaneous Xe-133 and Na-24 clearances. *J. Clin. Invest.*, 43:1805.
15. Rhodes, B. A., Rutherford, R. B., Lopez-Majano, V., Greyson, N. D., and Wagner, H. N., Jr. (1972): Arteriovenous shunt measurements in extremities. *J. Nucl. Med.*, 13:357.
16. Kakkar, V. (1972): The diagnosis of deep vein thrombosis using the ^{125}I fibrinogen test. *Arch. Surg.*, 104:152.
17. Lee, B. Y., and Trainor, F. S. (1977): Arterial flow in the lower leg correlated with plasma levels of two formulations of papaverine-hydrochloride. *Angio.*, 29:310.
18. Winsor, T. (1971): Vascular aspects of thermography. *J. Cardiovasc. Surg.*, 12:379.
19. Yao, V. S. T., Hobbs, J. T., and Irvine, W. T. (1969): Ankle systolic pressure measurements in arterial disease affecting the lower extremities. *Br. J. Surg.*, 56:676.
20. Winsor, T. (1950): Influence of arterial disease on the systolic blood pressure measurements in arterial disease affecting the lower extremities. *Am. J. Med. Sci.*, 220:117.
21. Strandness, D. E., Jr., and Bell, J. W. (1965): Peripheral vascular disease: Diagnosis and objective evaluation using a mercury strain gauge. *Ann. Surg.*, 161 (4):1.
22. Strandness, D. E., Jr., and Bell, J. W. (1964): An evaluation of the hemodynamic response of the claudicating extremity to exercise. *Surg. Gynecol. Obstet.*, 119:1237.
23. Johnson, W. C. (1975): Doppler ankle pressure and reactive hyperemia in the diagnosis of arterial insufficiency. *J. Surg. Res.*, 18:177.
24. Heyman, A., Karp, H. R., and Bloor, B. M. (1957): Determination of retinal artery pressure in diagnosis of carotid artery occlusion. *Neurology*, 7:97.
25. Fronek, A., Johansen, K. H., Dilley, R. B., and Bernstein, E. F. (1973): Noninvasive physiologic tests in the diagnosis and characterization of peripheral arterial occlusive disease. *Am. J. Surg.*, 126:205.

26. Rutherford, R. B., Hiatt, W. R., and Kreutzer, R. W. (1977): The use of velocity wave form analysis in the daignosis of carotid artery occlusive disease. *Surgery*, 82:695.
27. Barnes, R. W., Bone, G. E., Reinertson, J., Slaymaker, E. E., Hokanson, D. E., and Strandness, D. E., Jr. (1976): Noninvasive ultrasonic carotid angiography: Prospective validation by contrast arteriography. *Surgery*, 80:328.
28. Gosling, R. G. (1976): Extraction of physiological information from spectrum analysed Doppler-shifted continuous wave ultrasound signals obtained noninvasively from the arterial system. *IEE Med. Elec. Monograph for P. Peregrinus*, Stevenage, U.K., 21:73.
29. Barnes, R. W., Clayton, J. M., Bone, G. E., Slaymaker, E. E., and Reinertson, J. E. (1977): Supraorbital photo-pulse plethysmography: Simple accurate screening for carotid occlusive disease. *J. Surg. Res.*, 22:319.

Noninvasive Techniques for Assessment of Atherosclerosis in Peripheral, Carotid, and Coronary Arteries, edited by Thomas F. Budinger, et al. Raven Press, New York 1982.

Image Quality and Exposure Measurement in Diagnostic Ultrasound

*Paul L. Carson

University of Colorado Medical Center, Denver, Colorado 80220

The limitations and potential capabilities of ultrasound systems for assessment of atherosclerosis may be learned by measuring the data they produce against the ultrasonic interaction coefficients of tissues in the relevant anatomical regions. Clinical trials to validate system performance are essential at various stages of development, and even subjective, periodic evaluation of images from patients is essential.

EVALUATION OF SYSTEM PERFORMANCE

Performance Evaluation Techniques

In the past few years, considerable progress has been made in developing apparatus for accurate ultrasound system performance evaluation and in reaching agreement on useful procedures. Much of the newer equipment uses materials that simulate closely the ultrasonic interactions of the tissues to be studied, but electronic measurements and acoustic measurements in water are still the most appropriate for many purposes.

For pulse echo instrumentation, the following general characteristics should be documented using reproducible and preferably standard procedures: (a) ultrasonic frequency and bandwidth; (b) calibration and effects of system sensitivity controls; (c) signal:noise ratio, relative sensitivity of display modes, and uniformity of array response; (d) geometric resolution; (e) display characteristics of relative signal amplitude (time/range-dependent and time-independent); (f) geometric accuracy within image plane; and (g) delineation of scan plane. These characteristics are discussed in a draft document (1) that is perhaps the most complete and up-to-date discussion of precise performance evaluation measurements for pulse echo equipment. Standard methods for obtaining many of these performance evaluation measurements in detail

---

*Present address: Department of Radiology, University of Michigan Hospitals and Medical School, Ann Arbor, Michigan 48109.

are being published by user groups around the world. In particular, the American Institue of Ultrasound in Medicine (AIUM) has developed a standard method (2) for this most important aspect of measurement. The AIUM's draft standard on transducer performance (3) is to be submitted for publication in the next few months, and their article on the standard 100 mm test object (4) includes several useful, precise measurements as well as an essentially complete set of quality control tests. The International Electrotechnical Commission's (IEC) draft standard on performance evaluation of ultrasonic equipment is nearing acceptance, although in a form somewhat revised from their published discussion document (5). This standard includes several methods of measurement, allowing compliance with more specific national standards or practices. It emphasizes methods that do not require expensive equipment or extensive knowledge of electrical systems and covers many important performance evaluation concepts developed in the past few years.

Performance evaluation of Doppler equipment has been limited almost entirely to testing by its developers using a large variety of techniques. IEC's recent draft document on performance measurement of continuous-wave Doppler equipment is a bold step toward independent assessment—a usable, comprehensive set of standard Doppler performance measurements (6). Research groups having the appropriate personnel should adopt these procedures and develop the requisite phantoms, including tissue equivalents. This will speed universal acceptance of such procedures by prompting necessary modifications of them, assuring their accuracy and relevance. Extension of the concept to Doppler systems featuring range resolution should be pursued vigorously.

Performance Evaluation in Particular Applications

Physical performance measurements using various types of ultrasound equipment need to be closely correlated with their performance in specific applications. Appropriate *in vivo* measurements should be made in order to learn the systems' characteristics and limitations. Such performance should be determined by quantitative acoustic and geometric measurement in the body and by objective (or at least subjective) assessment of image quality and other criteria using an appropriate number of normal and pathologic cases or substituting phantoms designed to reproduce meticulously the acoustic properties of the relevant anatomy. In attempting to image coronary arteries, for example, it would be useful to determine the maximum acoustic path length for various transducer locations and the associated optimal frequency for imaging. It might be wiser to settle for usable results from arterial branches close to the transducer than to attempt imaging of more distant branches.

The amplitudes of echoes from the pericardium and other interfaces should be documented in an appropriate geometry to determine which levels in the lateral beam profiles and pulse waveform are limiting resolution of the vessels. By using tissue-equivalent substitutes to simulate the relevant anatomy, a great deal can be learned about the acoustic properties of the anatomy and attendant limitations on system performance. This may prove to be an excellent method of rapid quality assurance testing as well.

Careful system performance evaluation is practically useless if the information obtained is not wisely used. New medical research that is highly dependent on instrumentation always involves a choice between performance of clinical studies using still-evolving equipment and delay of the studies while equipment reliability and quality are being improved. Before beginning extensive clinical trials, which will only require repetition using better equipment in the near future, the design and physical performance of the instruments chosen should be carefully measured against state-of-the-art as well as potential alternatives.

Quality Assurance

Quality assurance tests should be performed regularly throughout the lifetime of clinical and research equipment. Either of two approaches (or preferably a combination of the two) is recommended: simplified quantitative tests (as with the AIUM standard 100 mm test object) or subjective evaluation and comparison of images from a tissue-equivalent phantom at fixed settings against previously recorded and stored images. Table 1 presents a list of quality assurance tests for pulsed echocardiography and their recommended frequencies of performance (7).

SAFETY CONSIDERATIONS AND MEASUREMENTS

Safety Factors and Their Relation to Information Content

It is extremely unlikely that ultrasound as commonly employed for diagnosis will ever cause significant harm to the patient or operator. Ultrasound is rightfully

TABLE 1. *Echocardiography quality assurance schedule[a]*

Maintenance function or test	Real-time arrays used frequently	M-mode units used frequently
Distance/time calibration error	W	SM
Sensitivity and uniformity		
Standard transducer	W	SM
Common transducers	SM	SM
All transducers	—	A
Axial resolution		
Standard transducer—3 FOVs	SM	SM
Common transducer—FOV	SM	SM
All transducers— 1 FOV	—	A
Photography and other hard		
copy recording	D	D
Lateral resolution, standard		
transducer	W	A
All transducers	SM	A
Check film processor quality		
control	—	—
Filters	SM	SM
Electrical and mechanical check	W	SM

[a]D, daily; W, weekly; SM, semimonthly; A, annually.

considered to be safer than diagnostic techniques using ionizing radiation, although it certainly has not been proved that it is safer under all diagnostic exposure conditions than the lowest-exposure X-ray procedures.

It is important, furthermore, not to consider diagnostic approaches like ultrasound as second-rate compromises chosen for their noninvasiveness at the expense of state-of-the-art performance. In many applications, ultrasound is known to provide the most complete and reliable information possible.

Tests of image quality and other criteria as a function of exposure conditions have been performed, but their results are not as refined nor as widely applicable as those from X-ray imaging tests. Ultrasound is much more complex and less well understood than X-radiation. Exposure conditions as a function of time and space vary widely among various applications of the several general and special modes of instrumentation for a given application. In many cases, system performance has not been raised to its theoretical best possible quality of exposure-limited performance, a particular handicap in special applications.

Furthermore, the relationship between modes of potential harm and the spatial and temporal distribution of the various ultrasound field parameters is relatively complex. In contrast, one may assume with reasonable assurance of accuracy that the effect of X-radiation is predictably cumulative, a simple function of the total energy absorbed at the site.

Regarding bioeffects, the system designer must ask: Under which conditions are we closer to the safety limits as defined by temporal *average* intensity (time-averaged power/unit of area), and when are these risks the greatest as measured by temporal *peak* intensity? In the past several years, it has been assumed that the thresholds most closely approached are usually those for thermal bioeffects. These effects are reasonably calculable functions of intensity averaged over the repetition period of the waveform and calculated as a function of exposure duration and spatial variables. The potential effects of mechanical stress and cavitation, however, also may be significant. Resonant oscillations of small air bubbles in the ultrasound field are receiving particular attention in light of their great potential as a contrast agent for ultrasonic imaging and for cardiovascular and other measurements.

Documentation of Exposure Conditions

While designing and using ultrasound systems as intelligently as possible, given the current state of knowledge, those planning and conducting research should provide for documentation of their exposure and performance characteristics. It is hoped that this would allow for individual judgment as to the level of detail and precision needed in various test situations. An interim standard (to be published) should aid considerably the definition of necessary exposure information and measurement of exposures (8). Manufacturers are expected to provide the exposure information required in this standard, which is intended to help researchers using commercially available equipment or equipment with similar characteristics.

REFERENCES

1. Carson, P. L., Zagzebski, J. A., et al. (1980): Pulse echo ultrasound instrumentation: performance evaluation and criteria. AAPM Report #8, American Association of Physicists in Medicine, New York.
2. American Institute of Ultrasound in Medicine (1979): AIUM standard specification of echoscope sensitivity and noise level including recommended practice for such measurements. *Reflections,* 5:1.
3. American Institute of Ultrasound in Medicine (1982): Standard methods for testing single element pulse echo ultrasonic transducers. AIUM. Chevy Chase, Maryland.
4. American Institute of Ultrasound in Medicine (1975): AIUM standard 100 mm test object and recommended procedures for its use. *Reflections,* 1:74.
5. Brendel, K., Filipczynski, L. S., Gerstner, R., Hill, C. R., Kossoff, G., Quentin, G., Reid, J. M., Saneyoshi, J., Somer, J. C., Tchevnenko, A. A., and Wells, P. N. T. (1977): Methods of measuring the performance of ultrasonic pulse-echo diagnostic equipment. *Ultrasound Med. Biol.,* 2:343.
6. Reid, J. M. (incorporating drafts by P. N. T. Wells and R. Gerstner): Methods of measuring the performance of continuous wave ultrasonic Doppler diagnostic equipment (draft). *(Personal communication).*
7. Carson, P. L., and Dubuque, G. L. (1979): Ultrasound instrument quality control procedures, Report 3: Center for Radiological Physics Report. American Association of Physicists in Medicine, New York.
8. American Institute of Ultrasound in Medicine (AIUM) and National Electrical Manufacturers Association (NEMA) (1979): AIUM-NEMA draft safety standard for diagnostic ultrasound equipment. Draft V, AIUM. Chevy Chase, Maryland.

Noninvasive Techniques for Assessment of Atherosclerosis in Peripheral, Carotid, and Coronary Arteries, edited by Thomas F. Budinger, et al. Raven Press, New York 1982.

Intravenous Angiography Using Digital Video Subtraction

Theron W. Ovitt, M. Paul Capp, Peter C. Christenson, H. Donald Fisher III, Meryll M. Frost, Sol Nudelman, Hans Roehrig, and George Seeley

Department of Radiology, University of Arizona Health Sciences Center, Tucson, Arizona 85721

We are developing an X-ray system that can image major arteries after the intravenous injection of radiocontrast dye. The image acquisition system consists of a high quality X-ray image intensifier-video chain. Images appear at the rate of one frame/sec, are converted into a digital format via an analog-to-digital converter, and are stored on a digital disc. Images made before the arrival of the radiocontrast material are then subtracted from those obtained after, so that the resultant image contains contrast only. The image is then electronically contrast-enhanced, and the final view of the arterial structures is displayed on a screen.

Carotid and renal artery images of diagnostic quality have been acquired from patients after validating the procedure with carotid and renal arteries and the heart in animals.

DESCRIPTION OF SYSTEM IMAGE ACQUISITION CHAIN

The image acquisition system is outlined in Fig. 1, which shows the major components as assembled in the experimental laboratory. A high-flux, high-heat-load X-ray source is required, since calculations indicate that a 1 mR exposure to the intensifier face is needed to detect 2% contrast levels in 1 mm structures. At present, exposures have been performed at only 0.4 to 0.5 mrad due to generator limitations. For examination of small arteries, however, the image intensifier must be capable of accepting a 1 mrad exposure without significant loss of resolution or contrast. The only intensifier we tested that meets this requirement is the new Phillips 14″ model.

The video system consists of an Amperex "frog's head" plumbicon incorporated into a Sierra camera and optically coupled to the image intensifier. Its most important feature is a high signal output of 2.5 to 3 A, with a preamplifier noise of 1 to 2 Na at a 5 MHz video band width, so that the signal:noise ratio is in excess of 800:1.

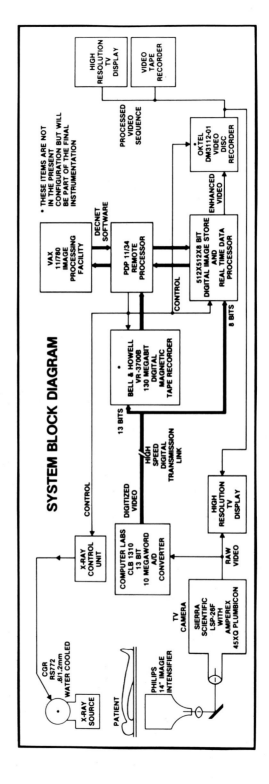

FIG. 1.

The A-to-D converter is a high-speed instrument capable of 10 megawords/sec with a 13-bit accuracy rate. This allows us to digitize in real time with 512 × 512 pixels, and to trade off improved resolutions for slower raster rates as needed. At present, we are utilizing only eight bits due to storage limitations of the digital image.

Our digital image store is a 512 × 512 × 8-bit charge-coupled device memory built in our lab. (This is soon to be expanded to a 2048 × 2048 display with up to 16 quantization levels.) It also has a mapping memory that allows any portion of the 256 gray levels to be expanded or compressed on the cathode ray tube (CRT) display. This gives considerable contrast enhancement to the displayed image.

The computer we use is a VAX 11/780 model, chosen for its relatively high utilization capabilities. Digitized images can be obtained at one frame/sec and stored within the computer as presently formatted. Any image can be subtracted from any other image and redisplayed on the CRT within 1 to 2 sec; both binary and logarithmic subtractions are conventionally performed. An Oktel video disc recorder is incorporated into the system for dynamic display as well as freeze frame scrutiny.

We are adding a Bell and Howell digital magnetic tape recorder to the system. When this is completed, 512 × 512 × 13 bits of raw data at 30 frames/sec or 1024 × 1024 × 13 bits of raw data at 7½ frames/sec can be instantly acquired and stored. This will allow complete post-processing of the data.

RESULTS

Our studies to date have produced excellent views of the carotid and renal arteries, the aorta, and left ventricular function in dogs. Coronary arteries have also been imaged in dogs, although not in their entirety.

This progress has allowed us to use intravenous angiography as the primary X-ray examination in studying extracranial carotid circulation in patients for whom carotid catheterization is too risky. These patients are usually elderly, and many have significant heart disease. We have performed 12 such examinations to date, all with satisfactory results.

Figure 2 shows an example of our studies. Fig 2a is an image obtained before antecubital injection of 50 cc Renografin-76 radiocontrast dye through a 16-gauge angiocatheter at 20 cc/sec. Figure 2b shows the unsubtracted image, with dye in the arterial structures, and Fig. 2c the subtracted image of 2a from 2b, clearly demonstrating the dye-filled carotid arteries. A slight motion of the patient's head is evidenced by the white, linear-streaked artifacts. Figure 2d shows the contrast-enhanced image of 2c.

DISCUSSION

The success of intravenous angiography depends on the following three factors: (a) The subject must be motionless for satisfactory subtraction—this requires alert, cooperative patients; (b) Enough contrast dye must be delivered to allow viewing of the arterial structures, even after the considerable physiologic dilution that always

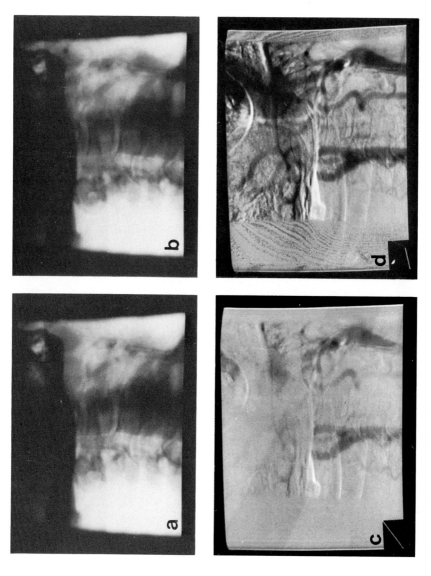

FIG. 2. First clinical demonstration of carotid arteries via intravenous angiography. **a:** Image of patient's neck before intravenous injection of contrast dye (50 cc Renografin 766). **b:** Image of patient's neck with contrast dye in arteries. **c:** Image obtained by subtracting **a** from **b**. **d:** Contrast dye enhancement of image **c**.

occurs; and (c) The X-ray system must be capable of delivering 0.5 to 1.0 mrad to the intensifier face; this will provide sufficient flux to discern low-contrast arterial images.

The results of both animal experiments and patient treatment indicate that these conditions can be met, and we anticipate that modification of our electronic imaging technique will minimize or eliminate motion problems. Our calculations indicate that subtracting two iodine-containing images (one image obtained at a kV energy slightly higher than the K-edge of iodine, the other immediately thereafter at a substantially higher kV) will produce a good contrast image even in the presence of minor-to-moderate motion. Validation of this theory awaits the incorporation of a rapid switching system in our X-ray generator.

The impetus for developing such a system was the need to detect and quantify atherosclerotic lesions in asymptomatic but high-risk patients. It is very difficult to assess atherosclerotic lesions in the human arterial system without angiography, unless the lesions are so severe that secondary effects occur. These include high blood pressure, angina, transient ischemic attacks, and (too often) more serious sequelae, such as stroke or myocardial infarction. Significant atherosclerotic lesions need to be identified *before* they cause symptoms, so that appropriate prophylactic therapy can be instituted. Because direct angiography is an invasive procedure requiring hospitilizazion, it is not feasible for identifying atherosclerotic lesions in the asymptomatic patient. The intravenous angiographic procedure was therefore developed as a screening method for latent but clinically important disease and for following patients serially to determine the effects of treatment on known atherosclerotic lesions.

One advantage of intravenous angiography is that it can be performed on outpatients, using a simple venous cannula rather than the more complicated arterial catheter. It is also a faster and thus potentially cheaper procedure (only 15 to 30 min/exam), and requires fewer personnel than angiography. However, angiography with arterial catheterization does have the advantage of higher resolution imaging that is not significantly degraded by patient motion or overlapping vessels. In comparison with ultrasound exams, furthermore, our system is not a completely noninvasive procedure. The radiation used, although in diagnostic amounts less than in standard angiography, makes it a potential hazard—even in patients beyond the childbearing age. Finally, the risk of allergic reaction to iodinated intravenous contrast dye, although small, is present.

In view of its initial success, intravenous angiography should become the primary examination of choice for evaluating large vessel disease in the aorta, carotids, renal and iliac arteries. Left ventricular function in wall motion kinetics should be easily seen using this technique, but this will have to await the incorporation of our aforementioned high-speed digital magnetic tape recorder, which will allow an image acquisition rate of up to 60 fields/sec.

Our ultimate goal is to visualize the coronary arteries in detail in order to identify coronary disease. Thus, instrumentation has accordingly been designed to image clearly a 50% stenosis in a 2 mm artery at a 2% contrast level. However, because of the shadows seen in cardiac chambers, visualization of coronary arteries will be difficult and will probably require additional image processing.

Noninvasive Techniques for Assessment of Atherosclerosis in Peripheral, Carotid, and Coronary Arteries, edited by Thomas F. Budinger, et al. Raven Press, New York 1982.

Intravenous Angiography Using Computerized Fluoroscopy Techniques

C. A. Mistretta, R. A. Kruger, D. E. Ergun, C. G. Shaw, M. Van Lysel, C. Strother, A. B. Crummy, J. F. Sackett, W. Zwiebel, D. Myerowitz, W. Turnipseed, and H. Berkoff

Department of Radiology, Clinical Science Center, University of Wisconsin, Madison, Wisconsin 53792

During the past few years, we have reported on preliminary imaging results using several time and energy subtraction algorithms implemented by a specially constructed real time digital image processor (1–6). Following extensive testing in animals, this device was interfaced to an image intensified fluoroscopy room in our Radiology Department. This chapter will describe the apparatus briefly and summarize what we have learned during the course of imaging 42 patients in the first 2½ months following installation.

Video fluoroscopy data are logarithmically amplified and digitized to eight bits/pixel with up to 512 pixels/line. Data are stored in any of three $256 \times 256 \times 13$ bit memories. These memories may be configured in several ways, depending on the particular imaging application. In all imaging modes, fully processed images appear during X-ray exposure and are stored on video disc or video tape at rates up to 60 images/sec. In cases involving significant patient motion, post-processing is sometimes required.

Perhaps the most promising application has been that involving imaging of the extracranial carotid arteries. Typically, a number 16 angiocath is inserted into the basilic vein in the antecubital region. Then, following injection of 30 to 40 cc of contrast agent, such as Renografin 76 or Conray 400, and a similar amount of saline flush, all injected at 15 to 20 cc/sec, a 0.25-sec X-ray exposure is made, and 16 television fields are integrated to form a 12 bit mask image. A few seconds later, as the carotids begin to opacify, a series of four field exposures (¹⁄₁₅ sec) are used to provide a 10 bit subtraction image at a rate usually chosen to be 1/sec. Examples of carotid images are shown in Figs. 1–3.

The sequence of several images is not as important in terms of the dynamics of the carotid filling as it is in overcoming artifacts due to patient motion. In most cases, movement of the spine can be accommodated by choice of an alternate mask image. A more serious artifact may be caused by swallowing. This motion is more complicated than that of the spine.

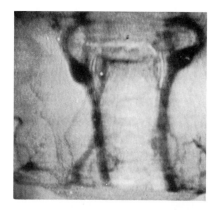

FIG. 1. Carotid arteries in AP projection following 40 cc Conray 40 injected at 14 cc/sec.

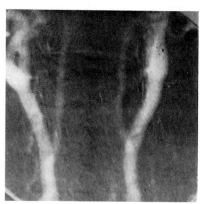

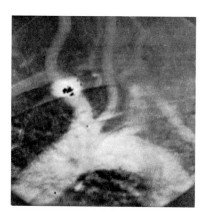

FIG. 2. **Left:** AP projection of carotid and vertebral arteries (40 cc Renografin 76, 40 cc saline). **Right:** A digital artifact appeared due to control switch in the wrong position (40 cc Renografin 76, 40 cc saline).

At present, our technique involves one anteroposterior (AP) and two oblique projections. In the AP, the swallowing artifact lies between the carotids and does not affect the image. However, in many cases, the AP projection does not show the carotid bifurcations clearly enough, so oblique projections are usually necessary. In the oblique projection, one carotid usually appears over the spine and the other lies over the throat. The one over the spine can almost always be imaged adequately. If there is no swallowing, a third projection may not be necessary. If there is, the second oblique projection is used.

The spatial resolution of our images is presently limited by our focal spot (0.6 mm) and our pixel density (512 × 256). The exposure for carotid imaging was chosen such that our quantum noise is somewhat larger than our system electrical noise. Typically, we run at 55 KVP, 240 ma with 5 mm of aluminum filtration. Under these conditions, the mask image requires an input patient exposure at the

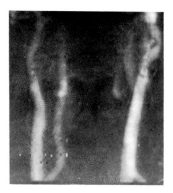 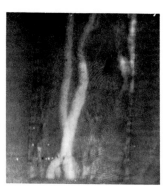 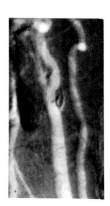

FIG. 3. AP and two oblique projections on the same patient. (All injections used 40 cc Renografin 76 40 cc saline flush.) There is an occlusion of the right external carotid artery.

back of the neck of about 400 mR. Each post-opacification ($\frac{1}{15}$ sec) image requires an additional 100 to 150 mR.

At this point, we have not yet compared this technique with angiographic and surgical results. We plan a study in 200 patients and hope to begin this as soon as we have implemented a number of improvements designed to increase the spatial resolution of our apparatus.

The technique has also been used to define the position of intracranial carotid arteries in patients scheduled for transphenoidal resection of pituitary tumors. In this case, it is conceivable that the intravenous technique could obviate the need for conventional arteriography.

Figure 4 shows images that include the subclavian arteries. Figure 4 (left) was obtained in the first 2 weeks following installation of our apparatus and required a 60 cc injection obtained by simultaneous 30 cc hand injections into two antecubital veins. Figure 4 (right) reflects the image improvements obtained using a better injection technique (30 cc power injected at 15 cc/sec into a single basilic vein) and following reduction of electrical noise in our video preamplifier and logarithmic amplifier.

Except in the region of the heart, a similar technique can be used to image arteries anywhere in the body. Figure 5, obtained with a 65 cc injection, shows one of several images obtained in the region of the renal arteries. In this case, breathing and bowel motion may give rise to artifacts such as those on the left side of the image. Superposition of vessels may also confuse the image to some extent. However, especially with improved spatial resolution, the image contrast should be adequate for many purposes.

Figure 6 (top) shows a radiograph in which stenoses are evident in the right and left iliac arteries. The intravenous digital subtraction image in Fig. 6 (bottom) shows the right iliac following transluminal angioplasty. The stenosis in the left iliac, which did not undergo the same procedure, is still evident. Figure 7 shows a graft in a femoral artery following a 72 cc intravenous injection.

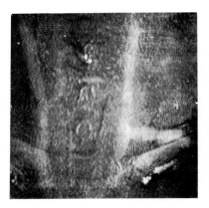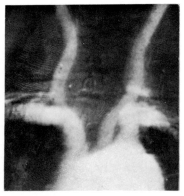

FIG. 4. Improvement in image quality due to revised injection technique and reduction of electrical noise in television preamplifier and logarithmic amplifier. (Some variation due to the different patients may also be present.) **Left:** October 1979—60 cc Conray 400, 30 cc hand injected into each of two basilic veins. **Right:** December 1979—30 cc single arm power injection at 15 cc/sec.

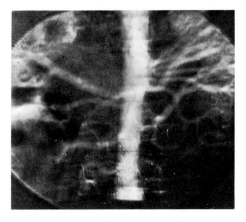

FIG. 5. Abdominal arteries following 65 cc (Renografin 76) plus 35 cc flush. Glucagon was not administered. Some bowel artifacts appear on the left of the image.

The heart poses far more difficult imaging problems than do the relatively fixed arteries discussed so far. The imaging tasks may be divided into three levels of difficulty: (a) real time left ventriculography; (b) imaging of coronary bypass grafts; and (c) imaging of coronary arteries. The first may be accomplished using injection of the order of 30 cc, provided that respiration can be suspended about 10 to 15 sec. In this case, a 60 field/sec image sequence can be subtracted from a preinjection mask, which is blurred by averaging over the heart cycle. This provides sufficient cancellation of anatomical background to permit iodine contrast to be amplified by a factor of about 8 relative to the conventional unprocessed fluoroscopic video output.

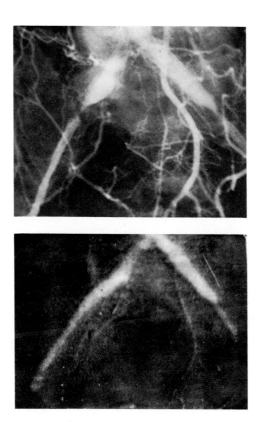

FIG. 6. Top: Arteriogram in region of iliac arteries. **Bottom:** Intravenous angiogram following transluminal angioplasty (72 cc Renografin 76 used).

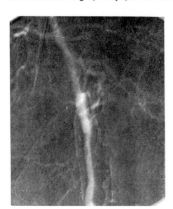

FIG. 7. Femoral artery graft following 65 cc injection with 35 cc flush.

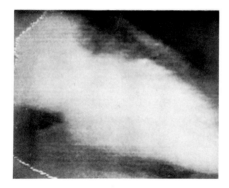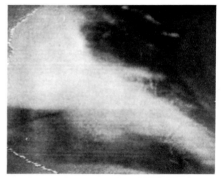

FIG. 8. **Left:** End diastolic left ventricle following 60 cc peripheral injection. **Right:** End systole.

Images of the left ventricle following a 50 cc injection are shown in Fig. 8. These images are best viewed as a dynamic display and are usually viewed using a video tape display.

In the event of patient respiratory motion, the image sequence may be reprocessed into our time-interval-differencing (TID) mode in which adjacent image intervals, separated by times that are short compared with the heart cycle, are sequentially subtracted from each other. This mode is relatively immune to motion artifacts and directly displays areas of dyskinetic motion as anomalous gray shades.

These techniques for left ventriculography have not as yet been systematically compared to alternative techniques, such as radioisotope imaging, angiography, or ultrasound. As far as quantitative measures, such as left ventricular (LV) ejection fraction, are concerned, the existence of the data in digital form may allow a determination of LV iodine content, which is independent of geometrical assumptions that are used in connection with angiocardiographic data. However, due to the use of an intravenous injection, the effects of overlapping contrast residuals in the right heart and lung field will have to be carefully considered.

We have studied several patients who had undergone coronary bypass surgery with the aim of assessing the patency of the grafts. Although we have not yet validated our observations in a controlled way, we have been able to gain some insights into the problems associated with this application. Because the exposure required for visualization of these grafts is greater than for visualization of ventricular wall motion, we have used two imaging modes designed to minimize exposure. In both modes, a preinjection mask is taken, so that gross anatomical structures can be subtracted. In the first mode, X-rays are pulsed for 10 to 15 msec during video camera blanking prior to video readout. This is repeated at a rate of 4/sec. The idea is to concentrate X-ray exposure into a few discrete images having good quantum statistical properties.

Primarily because of overlapping pulmonary vasculature, it has been difficult to analyze the grafts in these images. There is some possibility that use of ECG triggering to obtain a more completely registered mask would remove some artifacts generated by the moving opacified chamber boundaries, but in the right anterior oblique (RAO) and left anterior oblique (LAO) projections we have used thus far, the pulmonary vasculature and superposition of opacified left ventricle and aorta have been more serious problems. We intend to try weighted subtractions of images obtained just before left heart opacification in order to remove pulmonary effects. In addition, the AP and other projections will be tried in the hope of reducing overlap. Finding the best contrast injection rate and duration must also be carefully investigated.

The second method we have used for investigating bypass grafts is a dual dose rate procedure, in which a preinjection mask image is obtained using an X-ray tube current of about 300 ma. Then, following injection of contrast, low dose fluoroscopic subtraction is used to observe the passage of contrast through the right heart. When the left ventricle opacifies, the current is raised to 300 ma and three seconds of continuous subtraction images are obtained at a rate of sixty fields/sec (512×256). The exposure rate during this brief imaging sequence is usually somewhat greater than that used in conventional cardiac cineangiography. In spite of the need to review this brief sequence several times, we have had far greater success in identifying bypass grafts this way than by means of static images. Figure 9 shows a single subtraction image from the sequence just described. While some grafts, such as the left anterior descending (LAD) graft shown here, may be obvious, at least over part of its length, the characteristic motion of grafts is a great advantage for the purpose of distinguishing them from background structures, especially those in the lungs.

The TID mode discussed above may prove to be useful for assessing graft patency. In Fig. 10, subtraction images stored on a video disc during X-ray exposure were reprocessed to form image subtractions involving intervals ¼ sec apart. The object of this approach is to visualize the grafts because they have moved and to remove structures that are more stationary. In Fig. 10 (left), the origin of a right coronary graft can be seen near the surgical clips on the aorta. The more distal portion of the graft, which did not move in the chosen ¼ sec interval, is not seen. In Fig. 10 (right), a greater portion of the graft is seen. It should be mentioned that, in this

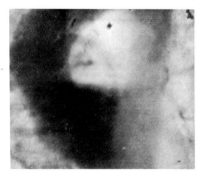

FIG. 9. Single image from dynamic subtraction fluoroscopy (60 cc Conray 400 used). The LAD graft can be seen under the aortic arch.

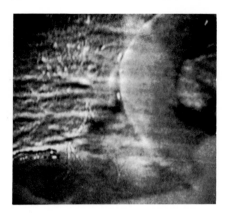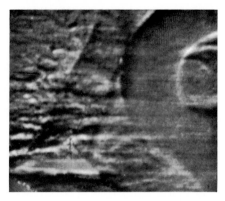

FIG. 10. **Left:** TID image showing origin of right coronary bypass and hints of two other grafts originating in the same area but poorly seen over the aorta. **Right:** Increased visualization of right coronary bypass graft (black). The other grafts now appear as black-white pairs.

mode, edge artifacts caused by the motion of larger structures, like the superior vena cava, can be mistaken for grafts. Also shown in Fig. 10 are two other grafts that originate at the aortic root and can be seen beneath the aortic arch.

The imaging of coronary arteries will be more difficult than the imaging of bypass grafts, which are larger and may be more easily projected away from the aorta. In our dog experiments, we were able to visualize the proximal portions of the major coronary arteries, again best perceived in a dynamic display. Since installation of our apparatus in our new hospital, we have not recognized coronary arteries in the bypass patients we have examined. These patients are obviously not ideal for such a procedure since, in most cases, the most easily visualized coronary segments have been bypassed. However, the problem of overlying pulmonary vasculature, which, so far, seems more serious than in our dog studies, and the concurrent opacification of the left ventricle and descending aorta may pose lasting problems even in normal patients.

We will reserve judgment on the question of whether or not coronary arteries may be visualized well enough to make any clinical difference until we have improved several imaging parameters, including exposure duration, focal spot size, recording medium, and our magnification, which is presently larger than optimal.

Aside from the question of coronary arteries, we feel that the technique involving real time digital processing of fluoroscopic video data following peripheral intravenous injection will be of certain use for evaluation of surgical results and for detection of major stenoses. The possibility of screening for early atherosclerotic disease, should the technique prove to be sufficiently reliable, will involve risk-benefit considerations of the somewhat elevated exposures required to form acceptable images in the presence of contrast concentrations diluted by a factor of 10 to 20 below those present in conventional angiography.

With regard to the instrumentation approach we have adopted, we are reasonably sure that the algorithms involved are sufficiently simple that the use of an expensive computer is not necessary and, in fact, usually will permit less flexibility and speed relative to a processor specifically dedicated to the generation and reprocessing of these intravenous angiograms. The ultimate value of the technique will be related to cost and simplicity. The approach we have taken can be provided as a relatively inexpensive accessory for almost any fluoroscopic X-ray room. The amount of interfacing for most applications can be implemented in a few days at most.

ACKNOWLEDGMENTS

Work supported by NSF Grant ENG 78-24555 and NSF Grant APR 76-19076, C. A. Mistretta, Principal Investigator, and by a General Research Support Grant to the University of Wisconsin Medical School from N. I. H., Division of Research Facilities and Resources.

REFERENCES

1. Kruger, R. A., Mistretta, C. A., Crummy, A. B., Sackett, J. F., Riederer, S. J., Houk, T. L., Goodsitt, M. M., Shaw, C. G., and Flemming, D. (1977): Digital K-edge subtraction radiography. *Radiology*, 125:243.
2. Kruger, R. A., Mistretta, C. A., Lancaster, J., Houk, T. L., Goodstitt, M. M., Riederer, S. J., Hicks, J., Sackett, J., Crummy, A. B., and Flemming, D. (1978): A digital video image processor for real time subtraction imaging. *Optical Engineering*, 17:652.
3. Kruger, R. A., Mistretta, C. A., Houk, T. L., Riderer, S. J., and Shaw, C. G. (1979): Computerized fluoroscopy techniques for noninvasive imaging of the cardiovascular system. *Radiology*, 130:49.
4. Houk, T. L., Kruger, R. A., Mistretta, C. A., Riederer, S. J., Shaw, C. G., and Lancaster, J. C. (1979): Real-time digital K-edge subtraction fluoroscopy. *Invest. Radiol.*, 14:270.
5. Kruger, R. A., Mistretta, C. A., Riederer, S. J., Ergun, D., Shaw, C. G., and Rowe, C. G. (1979): Computerized fluoroscopy techniques for noninvasive study of cardiac dynamics. *Invest. Radiol.*, 14:279.
6. Ergun, D., Mistretta, C. A., Kruger, R. A., Riederer, S. J., Shaw, C. G., and Carbone, D. (1979): A hybrid computerized fluoroscopy technique for noninvasive cardiovascular imaging. *Radiology*, 132:739–742.

Noninvasive Techniques for Assessment of Atherosclerosis in Peripheral, Carotid, and Coronary Arteries, edited by Thomas F. Budinger, et al. Raven Press, New York 1982.

Evaluation of Ischemic Heart Disease in Animals Using a Prototype Volume Imaging CAT Scanner

Erik L. Ritman

Departments of Physiology and Medicine, Biodynamics Unit, Mayo Foundation, Rochester, Minnesota 55901

Ischemic heart disease often involves localized stenosis of coronary arteries, a variable amount of collateral blood supply to the jeopardized myocardium, and reduced regional functional myocardial reserve. The disease decreases global cardiac function to a degree depending on total myocardial damage and somewhat on the site of the compromised myocardium. Multiple independent tests are commonly used to measure these four dynamically interacting manifestations. Such tests are usually performed at different times under varying physiological conditions, so that the relative importance of their results often remains open to question.

Recently, however, a minimally invasive method of testing for these conditions was introduced. The dynamic spatial reconstructor (DSR) X-ray imaging system can evaluate simultaneously all four manifestations of ischemic heart disease (Fig. 1). A prototype model of this multiple X-ray source computerized axial tomography (CAT) scanner was recently installed in our laboratory and is undergoing preliminary testing using animal subjects. It can simultaneously assess global cardiac function, coronary anatomy, regional myocardial perfusion, and total myocardial function by synchronous reconstruction imaging of the entire heart, including stop-action and rapid-repeat functions.

METHODOLOGY AND RESULTS

Coronary Artery Anatomy

A 15-kg dog was anesthetized, and tygon tubes from 0.6 to 3.2 mm in diameter were sutured to its epicardium following midsternal thoracotomy. The dog was scanned using 310 mg iodine/ml of roentgen contrast agent in the tubes.

The DSR correctly identified the locations of the tubes in each transverse image. The contrast agent appeared as bright spots, their sizes depending on the inside diameter of the tubing. Since the concentration of the agent was equal in all tubes,

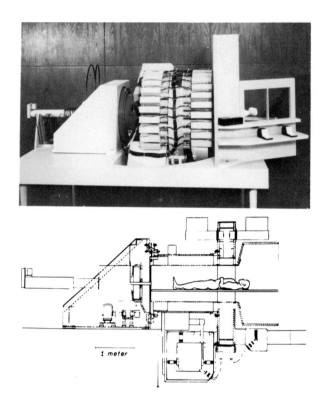

FIG. 1 *Upper panel:* A 1:5 scale model of the dynamic spatial reconstruction system recently installed at the Mayo Clinic's Medical Sciences Building. In this view, the array of 14 X-ray tubes is seen in the **lower half** and the opposing semicircular fluorescent screen and the associated 14 video imaging chains in the **upper half** of the circular gantry. **From left to right** are the slip ring assemblies for transmission of low-voltage power, logic, and video signals and high voltage and the stationary supporting structure housing the "X" bearing from which the rotating gantry is cantilevered. The gantry reveals most of the image chains; one of the 14 X-ray tubes is visible at the **lower aspect.** The large, −65 kV high voltage deck and smaller, high voltage, +65 kV bus bar enclosure are attached to the gantry on the **left** and **right** of the X-ray tubes, respectively. The head of a patient lying on the radiolucent table is seen through the window of the control booth. For cardiac scanning, the tabletop would be positioned further into the DSR "tunnel." The gantry will be separated from the patient area by a soundproof wall. The patient and clinicians would see only a stationary tunnel opening in one wall of the laboratory. *Lower panel:* Longitudinal section of the DSR system. Image-intensifier video camera chains, each similar to the highly successful, prototype single source dynamic spatial reconstructor, are positioned behind the fluorescent screen. The gantry will rotate (under computer control) around the cephalocaudal axis of the patient at a rate of 1.5°/$\frac{1}{60}$ sec over a full 360° (i.e., 15 rpm). A 10-msec, 162° circumferential electronic scan can be repeated at rates of up to 60 times/sec.

the brightness of the cross-sectional images of all tubes should theoretically have been equal. However, the images of the small diameter tubes were dimmer than those of the larger ones. In addition, these bright areas were larger than expected from the true tube diameters imaged. These blurring effects are probably due to the modulation transfer function characteristics of the imaging and reconstruction process.

The brightness $\times$ area product was then calculated for each tube. This figure is the sum of the CT scanner's X-ray density values (i.e., tube "CT" number minus heart wall "CT" number) for all voxels within the image of each lumen. The relationship between true tube lumen cross-sectional area and the brightness $\times$ area product computed from the images were linear over a tube lumen diameter range of 0.6 to 3.2 mm. The brightness $\times$ area product may be used to measure relative size for stenoses much narrower than permitted by the maximum spatial resolution capability of the DSR imaging system. The rationale for this index is that the total number of X-ray photons absorbed (and measured in cross section) by a tube filled with contrast agent determines the "total" brightness of its reconstructed image—even though this image is blurred (spread out) by the aforementioned modulation transfer function.

Transmural Blood Volume Dynamics

A 14-kg dog was anesthetized, and two atrial transeptal catheters were inserted with their tips in the left atrium. The heart was paced with a bipolar, right atrial pacing catheter. During the scan, 1 cc/sec of contrast agent (310 mg iodine/ml) was infused continuously into the left atrium. CT values in the subendocardial third, midwall third, and subepicardial third of the left ventricular free wall were sampled in each $\frac{1}{60}$-sec image throughout the cardiac cycle.

Transmural distribution of the left ventricular myocardial blood volume was indicated by the distribution of contrast agent (mixed with blood) in the coronary circulation. During the end diastolic phase of the cardiac cycle, the subendocardium was shown to be more opaque than the subepicardium—a finding consistent with published data suggesting preferentially increased subendocardial blood content in the normal heart. Subendocardial opacity (i.e., blood content) decreased more than subepicardial opacity during the early systolic phase. This observation suggests that subendocardial ischemia, a possible early sign of impaired coronary hemodynamics, is capable of detection.

Reduced Perfusion of the Region of Myocardium Supplied by a Ligated Coronary Artery

A 16-kg dog was anesthetized and its chest opened by left thoracotomy. The left anterior descending coronary artery was ligated about halfway between its origin and the apex of the left ventricle. During the subsequent scan, contrast agent was infused continuously into the aortic root via a catheter at a rate of about 2 ml/sec.

Reduced myocardial roentgen contrast agent in the reconstructed cross section of the heart was seen in a quite sharply demarcated region of the anterior free wall of the left ventricle that is ordinarily supplied by the ligated coronary artery. This indicates that the location and extent of regions of myocardium to which blood supply is interrupted by occlusion of a coronary artery may be clinically detectable following the injection of contrast medium.

Regional and Global Myocardial Function

A 15-kg dog was anesthetized and a thoracotomy performed on it. The left common coronary artery was cannulated and perfused with arterial blood from a larger, heparinized donor dog. The major vessels of the heart were ligated and divided, and the aorta and left atrium were cannulated and connected by a pumping circuit containing radiopaque medium (45 mg iodine/ml). Left atrial pressure and aortic outflow resistance were controlled.

This isolated heart preparation was suspended from the aorta, and the entire system could be rotated about the apex-to-base axis of the ventricle. This preparation maintained an output and pressure comparable to those normal for a denervated ventricle of similar size in the intact dog. Following a scan made under control conditions, the left circumflex coronary artery was ligated 2 cm distal to its origin, and the scan was repeated. The rate of systolic wall thickening and the thickness of the posterolateral free wall of the left ventricle, which is ordinarily supplied by this artery, were decreased.

To evaluate global ventricular function, total left ventricular myocardial mass and chamber volumes were calculated. This was achieved by identifying the endocardial and epicardial surfaces in each of the many parallel transverse images of the isolated ventricle and calculating the volume enclosed by each surface. Total left ventricular wall volume was found by subtracting the chamber volume from the volume contained within the epicardial surfaces. This procedure was performed once for each $\frac{1}{60}$-sec interval throughout one cardiac cycle. The resulting data allow calculations of end systolic, end diastolic, and stroke volume and—more importantly— wall dynamics in all regions of the myocardium.

Over the past decade, several clinical studies and animal experiments have suggested a direct relationship between the magnitude of regional myocardial blood flow and the percent and rate of regional left ventricular myocardial wall thickening during systole and wall thinning during diastole. The data we obtained using this working isolated left ventricle preparation are consistent with these study observations and indicate that the DSR can measure these parameters while assessing global cardiac function.

DISCUSSION

An important feature of the DSR system is that it presents data within 10 msec of the scan, thereby greatly limiting blurring due to movement and improving exact, beat-to-beat reproducibility of the shape, dimensions, and location of the heart required for gated CAT scanning. The DSR approach further allows retrospective computation of oblique and axial images without degradation of spatial and density resolution. Finally, the scan data produced by the DSR are formatted so that the thickness, exact location, and orientation of the slice can be superimposed perfectly on the lesion of interest, greatly increasing the utility of the image.

Of particular significance is the expectation that all the above DSR data will probably be obtainable using a single injection of contrast agent into the right ventricle or pulmonary artery. Assuming that at least 80 mg/ml of contrast agent are needed in the aortic root to opacify adequately the coronary arteries and myocardium, injection of at least 0.5 ml/kg is required. With the introduction of other high-speed, volumetric-imaging CAT scan machines with high-density resolution, perhaps a single injection of contrast agent into the right atrium or even into a peripheral vein may achieve these levels.

BIBLIOGRAPHY

1. Scanlan, J. G., Gustafson, D. E., Chevalier, P. A., Robb, R. A., Ritman, E. L. (1980): Evaluation of ischemic heart disease with a prototype volume imaging computed tomographic (CT) scanner: Preliminary experiments. *Cardiol.*, 46:1263–1268.
2. Ritman, E. L., Kinsey, J. H., Robb, R. A., Gilbert, B. K., Harris, L. D., and Wood, E. H., (1980): Three-dimensional imaging of the heart, lungs, and circulation. *Science*, 210:273–280.

Noninvasive Techniques for Assessment of Atherosclerosis in Peripheral, Carotid, and Coronary Arteries, edited by Thomas F. Budinger, et al. Raven Press, New York 1982.

Commentary

Alexander F. Metherell

Department of Radiology, South Bay Hospital, Redondo Beach, California 90277

I am very excited about the work described in the previous three chapters. I think that we are going to see a major advance in the practice of medicine come out of this work—in fact, it is going to revolutionize completely the way radiology is practiced.

I firmly believe that, in the next 10 years, we will move completely away from film-based radiography and into digital radiography, or electronic radiography—which is essentially what this is—for a number of reasons.

As you can see from these chapters, you can do things with electronic radiography that you cannot do with conventional film radiography. The technology has progressed to the point of applicability to ordinary film radiography (standard chest radiographs, for example).

This was not mentioned by the authors, but in addition to such conventional recording systems as the Bell & Howell models, a lot of companies are now designing optical disc recorders. The reason is that an optical disc can store between 10^{11} and 10^{12} bits of information in digital format.

I recently visited RCA and saw their prototype disc model in operation. It can record in digital format at a rate of about 30 megabits/sec. It allows you to digitize data from the CGR-16 or Phillips 14 models and, in real time, transfer those data onto an optical disc. The optical disc is about the size of a phonograph record and does not cost much more. With 10^{12} bits of information, if you split the radiography up, 1,000 by 1,000 pixels, just for mathematical convenience, you have 10^7 bits of information for each good-quality radiograph.

You can therefore store about 100,000 radiographs on one side of an optical disc, which costs less than $40. The cost of film, as you know, has been going up rapidly. Over the past year, there has been an increase of more than 100% in the cost of film, because the cost of silver is going up phenomenally.

As an example (because I want to make an economic point here), I understand that the hospital of the University of California in San Francisco had a film budget of $300,000 a year. It was $500,000 a year until they improved their quality control, but within a year that has doubled. You can see that their annual film budget, for a hospital of 600 or 700 beds, runs close to $1 million a year—not including the cost of the procedures themselves. Then they take all that money invested in film and store it in their film library.

If they keep 10 years' worth of film, which most large hospitals do, they have invested about $10 million. This is for only one large hospital, in the library, where it takes up a lot of space.

They could replace that file with approximately 30 videodiscs a year for less than $1,000. That is exciting to me, because I have an engineering background as well as a medical one. I can see the exciting potential of high technology being applied in the medical area. Medicine is becoming more and more technology dependent, and I think we need to approach that fact with an open mind. If we keep in mind cost-effectiveness, we will not have as much trouble gaining acceptance for high technology as we have had in the past.

I mention finances because in developing a complex technology like digital radiography, we stick our necks out. We can be criticized, as we were for CT development, which required such an expensive machine that Congress consequently passed laws requiring a certificate of need. We should be thinking constantly about the cost-effectiveness of such new systems, and I am convinced that it would be easy to demonstrate that these angiographic systems will prove extremely cost effective in medical health care delivery.

There is thus heavy economic pressure on manufacturers to develop digital electronic radiography. I am excited by this because, in the previous three chapters, we read of technology that is directly applicable to just about every area of radiology. That is going to revolutionize the practice of radiology.

This brings me to the subject that Dr. Richard Ross *(this volume)* introduced— technology transfer. He wrote in terms of tranfer of technology from the experimental phase into clinical use. However, there is another form of technology transfer that we should be considering, and that is technology transfer from one area of medicine to other areas of medicine.

Unfortunately, because the National Institutes of Health are so compartmentalized, we cannot examine anything here but atherosclerotic vascular disease. I think that some consideration should be given to mechanisms whereby technology that is developed in one small area in one of the Institutes can be rapidly disseminated to other areas within the Institutes. Technology transfer is thus an important consideration.

Obviously, if we want an angiogram of a patient, we are going to need a technology that will allow us to make it intravenously. Angiographic assessment can be done on an outpatient basis, however, whereas catheter techniques require a minimum of two days in the hospital. Again, we need such cost-effectiveness to meet certificate-of-need legislation.

I would like to propose some provocative ideas. Let us first focus on the goals of this volume.

The first goal to consider is to reach consensus on the potential of noninvasive techniques for detecting and quantifying plaques.

The second goal is plaque characterization. At the risk of being stoned, I am going to point out that angiography, including intravenous angiography, does not image plaques. Dr. Strandness (*this volume*) raised some questions about what we are seeing. Is it a calcified plaque, is it an ulcerated plaque, is it even a plaque? What is it?

What we are imaging is blood, or, more specifically, we are imaging the contrast material in the blood. By inference, when we look at the boundary wall, we say with our expertise, "That little squiggle there cannot be the normal boundary of a normal blood vessel; something else must be doing it, and with all my years of experience, I say it must be an ulcerated plaque." But we are not, in fact, looking at the plaque in angiography. When I thought about it, that bothered me, because I love all this beautiful technology. Let us not be discouraged, though, because for years and years, radiologists have been using angiography and diagnosing atherosclerotic plaques, and I think we need to keep that focused in our attention.

With respect to our first goal—the potential and problems of noninvasive techniques for detecting and quantifying plaques—I think we could argue that the angiographic techniques, be they catheter or intravenous, do allow us to detect and quantify plaques. At the moment, that is the gold standard for identifying plaques, but it is an indirect method. I want you to remember that.

The techniques that have been described do not satisfy the second goal, which is to determine the potential of noninvasive techniques for meeting the needs of plaque characterization. I think that they do not characterize the plaque because they do not look at the plaque itself—they look at the blood surrounding plaques.

Can these techniques be made to satisfy the second goal? I believe that potentially they can be. For example, we all know that CT has such contrast sensitivity that you can measure different tissue areas. If you are imaging a lipid area, you should be able to see it, because a calcified aorta screams at you from the TV screen on the CT scan. We know that X-rays are capable of doing this, but the way angiography is used right now, it does not directly image plaques.

Perhaps we should think about adapting X-rays to do this. The question is: Can we adapt the kind of system that Dr. Ritman wrote about, and could that system be used at sufficient spatial and contrast resolution to give specific information about what the plaque consists of? I think it can, but we have to pay the price of increased dosage. If we want better spatial or contrast resolution, then the CT dose has to go up.

Using the GE-8800 scanner, available everywhere, we can image the ophthalmic artery in the eye. If we can do that, surely we can modify the CT scanner to resolve coronary arteries and maybe parts of the coronary arteries. If we get good enough resolution, we may be able to see the plaque itself, not just the blood and the contrast material. That is the first step.

The next step goes beyond that: Do not use contrast. Do not inject anything, but improve the spatial and contrast resolution so that you can actually see the plaque itself.

I present these few ideas to you and leave you with these key words: technology transfer and cost-effectiveness.

Noninvasive Techniques for Assessment of Atherosclerosis in Peripheral, Carotid, and Coronary Arteries, edited by Thomas F. Budinger, et al. Raven Press, New York 1982.

Coronary Arteriography: An Invasive Art

Melvin P. Judkins

Department of Radiology, Loma Linda University Medical Center, Loma Linda, California 92350

Coronary angiography, properly performed with imaging in multiple projections, accurately depicts anatomical change and ventricular dynamics in the living. It is the gold standard by which every other imaging method must be measured. This does not imply, however, that coronary arteriography is the only useful imaging modality or that a better imaging method will not be developed in the future.

To visualize the coronary anatomy adequately, all major proximal parts of the coronary tree should be imaged in at least two planes in which the X-ray beam is at right angles to the vessel. The receptor should faithfully reproduce the input image. Each X-ray image must be produced by sufficient quanta to portray the vascular luminal anatomy accurately and suppress noise.

Multiple factors influence ventricular function; the fundamental and essential factor is patent plumbing. The coronary pipes provide fuel for cardiac muscular function. The coronary vessels themselves are dynamic and their anatomy or functional anatomy may change. A vessel severely stenosed or occluded today may be functionally patent tomorrow.

It has been shown that the highest degree of interpretive accuracy (about 90%) is achieved when several experienced readers view the subject simultaneously, discuss it, and arrive at a consensus. Prior knowledge of patient history predisposes to inaccuracy and missed lesions.

Accuracy of interpretation is directly related to quality of study. As the image quality deteriorates, interpretive accuracy declines. Interpretive difficulties are accentuated in noninvasive studies when the image being viewed is imprecise. Accuracy of diagnosis then is dependent on quality of image and expertise of consensus of interpretation.

In the future, imaging of coronary anatomy and ventricular function will be accomplished noninvasively with the accuracy of today's invasive studies. Reconstructed functional images will provide more information than is currently available to the cardiac surgeon at the time of operation and to the cardiac angiographer. Until that day, we must use the tools that we have to our greatest advantage.

Noninvasive Techniques for Assessment of
Atherosclerosis in Peripheral, Carotid, and
Coronary Arteries, edited by Thomas F.
Budinger, et al. Raven Press, New York
1982.

Commentary

Melvin P. Judkins

*Department of Radiology, Loma Linda University Medical Center,
Loma Linda, California 92350*

We must not overlook the importance of the history and the physical examination. When talking about noninvasive techniques, we immediately assume that anything that is noninvasive is angelic. Conversely, of course, an invasive technique is of the devil. I think invasive versus noninvasive is an invalid comparison. The important considerations are: What studies can be done, what can be ascertained, and for what price, both in dollars and cents and in mortality and morbidity.

Among our subspecialties we work together to provide patient care in various ways. I believe the best plan is a team approach and that it is very important we function as a real *team*, regardless of what our special interests may be. We should work toward the common goal of diagnostic excellence.

There are several methods of accomplishing this goal. The straightforward direction is the simplest and the fastest. At this symposium, we have considered different methods of arriving at the same point. Unfortunately, the thing that we have failed to recognize is that not only are there different methods of arriving at the same place, but there also may be slightly different results of pursuing different methods. For example, those who run the health care system say, "You must follow *our* prescribed plan to get the desired results." But theirs is not necessarily the best route. Sometimes we need to take others. More than one type of examination is very often indicated. The history is the first, and the physical examination the second. A group of tests, both noninvasive and invasive, may be required to supply the needed information and in the end, serve the patient best, probably with the least expense.

Let us consider a coronary artery image. Initially the vessels are only faintly visible. We add more data points (information) and there is a better image; additional data points allow us to better visualize the vessel. But there is still not enough information to produce an adequate image. We add still more data points and now there is a diagnostic quality coronary arteriogram. We can identify a lesion with confidence; we have valid information.

Sometimes needed information is obscure or partially hidden. We must be able to view anatomy in multiple projections. In one patient, the angled projection revealed a double coronary vessel lesion. Without this projection an erroneous diagnosis would have been made. One of the problems inherent in some noninvasive techniques is the inability to view structures in as many projections as needed to adequately depict the anatomy. An invasive technique sometimes is required to provide information needed for a definitive diagnosis.

At a crossroad in decision making, a choice must be made. The key question is, "For this patient, which examinations and techniques are proper to most accurately and expeditiously diagnose and treat his particular problem?" Our goal should be to obtain information that will provide all the facts and enable us to provide optimal individualized patient care.

Noninvasive Techniques for Assessment of
Atherosclerosis in Peripheral, Carotid, and
Coronary Arteries, edited by Thomas F.
Budinger, et al. Raven Press, New York
1982.

Full Capability Doppler Diagnosis in Extracranial Vascular Disease

Merrill P. Spencer, John M. Reid, and Donald L. Davis

Institute of Applied Physiology and Medicine, Seattle, Washington 98122

PRESENT CAPABILITY OF DOPPLER ULTRASOUND

Doppler ultrasonic detection of blood flow in the arteries was first used for extracranial cerebrovascular disease by Brockenbrough in 1956 to detect the changes in velocity of periorbital arterial signals. These techniques, refined and developed by others, have made an excellent contribution by detecting collateralization caused by hemodynamically significant carotid artery obstruction. They have a high sensitivity but have problems in specificity, since the obstruction must be sufficient to produce collateralization. Also, intracranial collaterals from the opposite internal carotid or from the vertebral arteries may diminish the apparent collateralization effect.

Other non-Doppler techniques for collateralization around the eye include indirect pressure measurements in the retinal artery, such as ophthalmodynamometry and cutaneous photoplethysmography. These techniques carry the same degree of accuracy as Doppler detection of collateralization and bear the same problems of Doppler. A serious disadvantage of all collateral techniques arises because they are indirect tests for obstruction and cannot separate a tight stenosis from total occlusion of the carotid artery.

Hand-held probing with the Doppler has also been applied successfully to detect obstructive disease of the vertebral artery and subclavian artery, and a highly accurate test has been devised for vertebral to subclavian steal. Subclavian stenosis and vertebral-subclavian steal are frequently found when routine Doppler examination of these arteries is employed. Most of these lesions are found in asymptomatic patients, but the clinical significance of vertebral steal can be disclosed by the use of a provocative test applying reactive hyperemia to the area of the affected side while maneuvering the patient from a reclining to a sitting position. If this maneuver

95

produces or exacerbates symptoms of vertebral-basilar insufficiency, the patient may benefit from surgery. Obstructions at the aortic origin of the innominate or left subclavian are diagnosed by downstream Doppler abnormalities of obstruction coupled with findings of bruits in the upper chest and neck.

Hand-held probing of the carotid arteries has also been developed by Gosling and by Pourcelot using pulsatility characteristics to diagnose carotid obstruction. Hand-held probing can rarely detect abnormalities within the actual stenosis.

Direct Doppler imaging of the carotid arteries at the bifurcation has been developed with both continuous wave (C-W) and pulsed Doppler ultrasound. With C-W, at least, it is possible to detect reliably and reproducibly high velocities up to 500 cm/sec within a stenotic lesion, as well as the secondary features of downstream turbulence, artery wall vibrations, and changes in pulsatility. C-W Doppler imaging can quantitate the degree of stenosis and separate tight stenosis from total occlusion. The accuracy of C-W Doppler to detect stenosis is greater than 90% when compared with X-ray angiography.

An important and unique capability of C-W Doppler imaging is the differentiation of grade IV and grade V stenoses from occlusion of the internal carotid. In patients with transient ischemic attacks, this differential diagnosis determines whether carotid endarterectomy will or will not be performed. This is a crucial clinical matter in stroke prevention—not from loss of the final threadlike lumen, which will not affect brain perfusion, but from occlusion, because of the danger of large emboli breaking loose from red fibrin clots forming downstream to the tight grade V stenosis.

Bifurcation imaging, when combined with periorbital and other hand-held examinations of the vertebral and subclavian system and used with auscultation and the clinical history, provides the basis for an integrated consultation report to the referring physician that exceeds the usefulness of single techniques alone (Davis). The complete cerebrovascular evaluation used in our laboratories is outlined in Table 1. C-W Doppler diagnoses of obstructive extracranial cerebrovascular lesions are illustrated in Fig. 1.

Nonstenotic plaques are also diagnosed because of the effect of calcium deposits in scattering the sound beam and producing abnormal Doppler signals. As the ultrasound beam traverses the arterial wall, scattering of the beam by calcium deposits or roughening of the lumenal surface produces recognizable features on the Doppler-shifted signals (Fig. 2). Recent *in vitro* studies of excised iliac arteries have confirmed that calcium deposits in atherosclerotic plaques can produce asonic gaps in the Doppler image and inverted signals. In addition to these features, if fluttering caused by localized turbulence is detected without the high frequencies of stenosis, a diagnosis of nonstenotic plaque can also be made. A diagnosis of intimal ulceration alone cannot be made by Doppler ultrasound.

A diagnosis of syphon stenosis can be made from the combination of findings of a bruit over the eye and a high pulsatility index in the internal carotid velocity pulse.

TABLE 1. *Outline of Doppler cerebrovascular evaluation*[1]

History
  Carotid insufficiency symptoms
  Vertebrobasilar symptoms
Physical examination
  Neurological survey
  Arterial palpation
  Thoraco-cephalic auscultation
  Arm pressures
Doppler examinations
  Doppler imaging
    Carotid bifurcation
    Subclavian-vertebral and low common
  Hand-held probing
    Ophthalmic artery signals
      Posterior orbital
      Periorbital
  External and internal carotid signals
  Vertebral artery signals
    Base of skull
    Anterior-supraclavicular
  Subclavian, axillary, and brachial signals
Diagnostic interpretations
  Carotid arteries
    Bifurcation—Stenosis and occlusion (of internal,
      external, or common)
    Aneurysm
    Collateral evaluation
    Plaquing without stenosis
  Vertebral arteries
    Stenosis
    Subclavian steal
  Subclavian and innominate arteries
    Stenosis and occlusion
  Cardiac
    Low output
    Arrhythmias
    Miscellaneous

[1]System of Spencer and Brockenbrough.

FUNDAMENTAL DOPPLER SIGNAL CHARACTERISTICS

The range of useful C-W Doppler audio characteristics of blood flow may be categorized according to location, amplitude, frequency, direction, and pulsations and is summarized in Table 2.

The *location* from which the Doppler signal is obtained is highly specific to a given vessel segment and, with pulsed Doppler, may be refined to velocity profiles.

The *amplitude* of the Doppler signal is the least reliable characteristic, because in the transcutaneous mode it depends on many factors that do not relate to blood velocity or blood flow, such as the distance of the blood vessel from the transducer, and intervening ultrasonic obstructions, such as air bubbles in the coupling jelly as

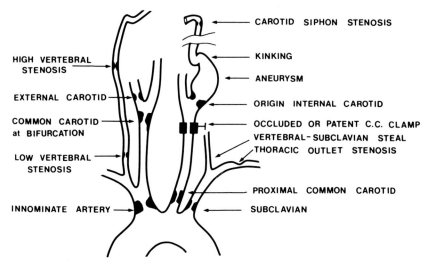

FIG. 1. Obstructive lesions of the aortocerebral circulation diagnosed by Doppler.

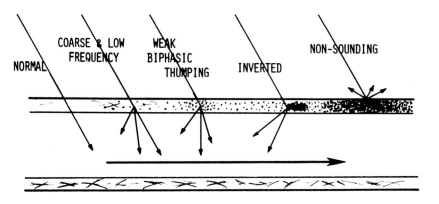

FIG. 2. Effects of calcium deposits on Doppler ultrasound.

well as the ultrasonic opacity of intervening tissues. Amplitude is useful, however, when used in conjunction with other abnormalities and when comparing symmetrical arteries of the body.

The *audio frequencies*, or more precisely the frequency spectrum of the Doppler signal, are the single most useful characteristics, particularly when following the signal along the axis of vessels running parallel to the body surface or comparing symmetrical arteries on opposite sides of the body and in following changes in frequency within the same artery and from one examination to the next. The spectral distribution carries information concerning mean and maximum velocity, turbulence, and plaquing.

TABLE 2. *Usable characteristics of Doppler signal*

Location	Specific vessel segment
Amplitude	Comparative information
Frequency	Velocity distribution
Pulsations	Resistance indices, diastolic component, acceleration
Direction	Pressure gradient, turbulence

The *direction* of blood flow is usually identified by direction-sensitive circuitry. Direction can change within the heart cycle and can be in both directions simultaneously in both normal and turbulent conditions. Pitfalls are occasionally caused by curvature of the artery direction or nearby bony structures. Bony structures or the presence of calcified plaquing within the artery wall may sufficiently scatter the sound beam that is reflected to produce inverted signals making the blood flow direction appear falsely reversed (Fig. 2).

Pulsations of the frequency spectrum within the cardiac cycle carry a great deal of physiological information for the interpreter who recognizes the underlying hemodynamic causes. The pulsatility index reflects the relative amount of diastolic runoff present and is related to the resistance of the outflow vasculature and arterial wall elasticity. Changes in the systolic acceleration of the blood flow provide a relatively unexploited characteristic. Slow acceleration indicates obstruction proximal to the point of examination.

Amplitude, frequency, pulsation, and direction characteristics of Doppler can be modified by mechanical compressions or pharmacological means to assist the examination and its interpretation. Carotid and temporal artery compressions have become a significant part of the complete periorbital and posterior orbital Doppler examination. The effect of carotid compression on vertebral signals at the base of the skull has only recently been devised in our laboratory to evaluate the collateral between the carotid and vertebral circulations.

Many audiovisual presentations of the Doppler signal characteristics are available to assist the interpreter. These include spectral display, analog tracings, and imaging. Using the human hearing mechanism by listening directly to the signal qualities, even without recording, is the single most useful method of analyzing and interpreting Doppler signals, because all signal characteristics are represented, including direction, if stereo speakers are used. The exact location of the signal, of course, is determined by the examiner. For clinical purposes, the human hearing-analysis mechanism exceeds electronic means of recognition of most characteristics. Instrumentation assists listening by selecting and quantitating special characteristics, such as mean velocity and velocity profiles, as well as dual-directionality of the signal. The advantages and disadvantages of listening, as well as the other methods of presentation, are outlined in Table 3.

In spite of the great amount of physiological and diagnostic information available on Doppler noninvasive evaluation of the circulation, the use of the Doppler tech-

TABLE 3. *Doppler audiovisual presentations*

Listening—All characteristics present
  Advantages
    Exceeds most electronic means for clinically significant
      features
    Faster interpretation
  Disadvantages
    Subjective, requires great skill
Spectral display—all characteristics present
  Advantages
    Objective, training aid, quantitative
    Makes the best of weak signals
  Disadvantages
    Additional cost, important qualities may not be recognized
Analog signal tracings
  Advantages
    Selected features objectively quantitated
  Disadvantages
    Sensitivity limited to strong signals
    Discards useful information
Doppler imaging
  Advantages
    Location of signal objectively quantitated allowing careful
      search of important vessel segments
  Disadvantages
    Requires more training
    More costly than hand-held technique

nique has spread slowly within the medical field. Only a few physicians willing to learn the necessary skills and understand the basic physiological principles have benefited from its availability. Undoubtedly, the limitations for many are related to the difficulties in understanding the audio presentation of the findings when most physicians are visually oriented. As a parallel example, audio information, such as auscultation of the heart, has traditionally been regarded as "soft" information and has been difficult to teach.

Recent availability of bidirectional color spectral display, the video format, and binaural dual direction audio signals provides the availability of a composite audiovisual display of all C-W Doppler characteristics simultaneously in a dynamically reproducible format. Simultaneous seeing and hearing of all the characteristics of Doppler in video format is now possible, and high-quality records can be made. The purpose of this chapter is to disclose a composite audiovisual display that presents all the information available in C-W Doppler in a video format for replay and objective illustration and interpretation.

COMPOSITE DOPPLER DISPLAY

The composite audiovisual display system is illustrated in Fig. 3. The bidirectional color spectral display was developed by. Dr. Ron Hileman and Mr. Joseph Cairo

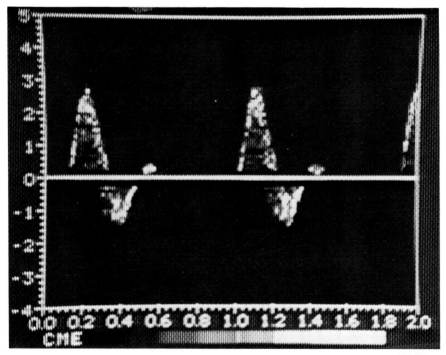

FIG. 3.

of Carolina Medical Electronics and uses a microprocessor single-board computer and Fast Fourier Transform with a 5 msec updating time. It operates on the phase difference between signals generated from motion toward and away from the ultrasound source. Blood velocities away from the probe are represented by frequencies above the zero baseline, while blood velocities toward the probe are represented by frequencies below the baseline.

Two selectable frequency scales are available, including either 0 to 5 kHz positive and 0 to 4 kHz negative or 0 to 10 kHz positive and 0 to 8 kHz negative. Three time bases are available, including full sweeps of 1, 2, or 10 sec. The amplitude of the audio frequencies is represented by a color coding. These amplitudes are represented on a thermal scale, with red representing the lowest and white the greatest amplitude. Oranges and yellows represent the middle signal directly displayable on a TV monitor and recordable on a video tape recorder. Figure 3 represents the directional and amplitude capability of this spectral display of signals recorded from the femoral artery of a normal human subject.

Dual direction audio signals from bidirectional Doppler are provided by use of the circuitry of Nippa, which cleanly separates forward flow (away from the transducer) from reverse flow (toward the transducer). The separate directional audio signals are recorded on the stereo channels of a video tape recorder and also presented on stereo speakers mounted on either side of the spectral display.

The carotid bifurcation image is displayed in a special insert on the spectrum display, as seen in Fig. 4. Voice annotations are preserved and are mixed with the forward flow signal. To preserve clean separation of the audio signals, the technician performs the examination with either a throat microphone or head set to listen to the Doppler signals on the voice channel.

By means of an insert window on the spectral display, the Doppler image of the carotid bifurcation is displayed. This is accomplished by a TV camera focused on the imaging oscilloscope, and through a split screen device, sharing of the video channel is accomplished. The exact position of the Doppler probe and the source of the audio signals are continuously provided for the interpreter. This probe position is indicated by a bright spot normally produced by the Doppler signal in image development. The bright spot serves as an automatic cursor for the source of the video displayed Doppler signals and the stereo speaker sounds.

From the video format, the maximum frequency is measured at any point in the beat cycle and can be used to determine the degree of stenosis by the methods previously disclosed by Spencer and Reid (*this volume*). In addition, the acceleration of the velocity pulse can be measured from the leading edge of the spectral display. This acceleration index can be measured in units of kHz/sec^2 or cm/sec^2. This measurement is accomplished from a straight line drawn tangent to the maximum slope of the velocity pulse. The acceleration is most accurately accomplished when the spectral sweep is in the 1 sec mode. Differences in acceleration between sym-

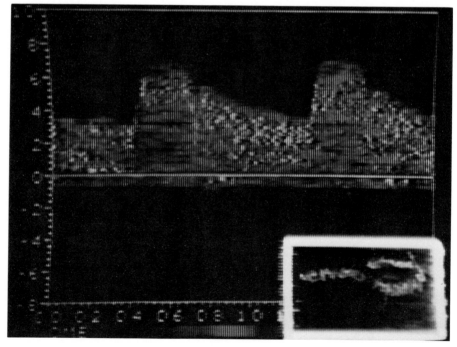

FIG. 4.

metrical signals from each side of the body are an index of the degree of the damping of the signal.

Evaluation of the new composite display was performed on routine patients passing through two of this Institute's vascular laboratories in Seattle, Washington, and on normal volunteers. In addition, audio tape recordings of patient examinations at the second vascular laboratory were "played" through the spectral analyzer and stereo speakers for further experience.

DISCUSSION

The value of the simultaneous display of all C-W Doppler characteristics is discussed in the following:

1. It increases precision of signal localization by indicating more accurately where the Doppler signals arise. (Previous imaging techniques grossly correlated the source of the signal by voice annotations from the technician.) This increased resolution: (a) increases separation of internal from external signals at the origin from the common carotid and increases accuracy in designating whether high frequencies of stenosis arise from the external, internal, or common carotid; (b) indicates to the interpreter the thoroughness with which the technician has searched the bifurcation area for diagnostic signals; (c) improves the morphological and physiological representations, such as the length of the stenotic segment and details of flow signals upstream and downstream to the stenotic lesion. Of special interest is the future possibility of visualizing "craters" in the arterial wall by identifying stable vortices; and (d) improves the differentiation of total occlusion of the internal from grade IV and grade V stenoses.

2. It improves quantitation of stenosis by: (a) indicating to the technician where the highest frequency is located and specifying its exact value. The maximum frequency, not always audible, is further apparent on the real-time spectrum display, visually indicating to the examiner when and where the maximum frequency occurs; (b) The maximum frequency can be immediately quantitated for accurate on-line diagnosis of the degree of stenosis using the established correlations of the signal frequency within the stenosis diameter; (c) The $f2/f1$ frequency ratio method of measuring the percentage of stenosis is improved in accuracy.

3. It encourages new clinics to use the capabilities of Doppler by: (a) simplifying the examination and interpretation techniques; and (b) providing training concerning the understanding of the audio signals.

The advantages of X-ray angiography over Doppler ultrasound are its superior morphology and the intracranial information that it provides. The advantages of Doppler over X-ray angiography are that it is safe and painless, is less costly, requires a shorter examination time, and provides superior functional information. In one sense, its morphology may actually be superior to X-ray. This is because the C-W Doppler signal represents the blood velocities within the entire cross section of stenotic arteries, unlike the X-ray, which is limited to a few projected diameters at best not accurate through ± 0.5 mm. Since plaques are usually asymmetrical, Doppler accuracy in skilled hands probably exceeds X-ray angiography.

Future additions to full capability presentations of Doppler will include an electrocardiogram (ECG) signal on the screen and automatic triggering of the spectral sweep from the R-wave of the ECG. This addition will allow comparisons of phase lags between signals. Also useful will be the inclusion of the ear pulse on the spectral screen when carotid compression is performed in order to confirm the adequacy of the compression. A probable future addition to the video presentation will be monitoring of the patient and probe position in the location window.

As effective medical and surgical treatment options unfold, methods of selecting patients who will benefit from a given treatment and management regime increase in importance. The use of noninvasive techniques and further understanding of the natural history of the atherosclerotic plaque will help identify the risk of stroke on both a statistical and individual basis. Noninvasive techniques will also be useful in proving the effectiveness of atherosclerosis prevention and resolution methods. The full capability of Doppler ultrasound toward these ends is now available through the composite video presentation presented here.

In the stroke prevention arena, the problem of differentiation of transient ischemic attacks due to carotid embolization from those attacks due to carotid insufficiency is paramount. Doppler ultrasound excels in detecting and quantitating stenosis of the carotids and subclavian vertebral obstructions. The Doppler image should be considered a method of localizing the physiological qualities. At the present time, Doppler cannot specify ulceration in terms of denuded endothelium.

In the future, the combined advantages of C-W and pulsed Doppler, as well as real-time imaging, may be accomplished by the infinite gate pulsed Doppler (IGPD). The IGPD provides velocity profiles of all vessels in its path at a rate of the pulse repetition rate. By providing both long and short time interval gates, the received signal can provide the ease of vessel finding inherent in C-W, and high resolution Doppler images can be provided by the short sample gate. By means of beam deflection techniques, sector scans can also be provided to accomplish real-time imaging. These multiple uses of the pulse require time sharing or other technology not yet applied to ultrasound.

Noninvasive detection of intimal ulceration and platelet and thrombus adherences to the artery wall is an important need in prevention of stroke. X-ray angiography, though it sometimes identifies deep craters, cannot specify denuded endothelium. The angiographic interpretation of "ulceration" is often dependent on clinical signs of transient ischemic attacks. Also, craters are often seen on the asymptomatic side when bilateral carotid angiography is performed. The greatest likely identification is of adherent thrombus, intimal flaps, and other flagging tissue threads within the artery lumen. The ultrasonic resolution necessary for these diagnoses may be near, but it is not now present in the commercial units generally available. A likely approach to noninvasive thrombus detection might use radioisotope tagging and detection techniques. These have found some usefulness in venous thrombosis, but they have not been developed sufficiently for the arteries.

Noninvasive Techniques for Assessment of
Atherosclerosis in Peripheral, Carotid, and
Coronary Arteries, edited by Thomas F.
Budinger, et al. Raven Press, New York
1982.

Pulsed Doppler Imaging of the Carotid Bifurcation

David S. Sumner

*Department of Surgery, Section of Peripheral Vascular Surgery, Southern Illinois
University School of Medicine, St. John's Hospital, Springfield, Illinois 62769*

In 1971, D. E. Hokanson, working in the laboratories of D. E. Strandness, devised a pulsed-Doppler imaging system for mapping the flow stream of peripheral arteries (1–3). The impetus for this research was the need for an accurate, noninvasive means of depicting the arterial lumen. Conventional B-mode scanning had been disappointing when used for this purpose, since its echoes did not reliably define the blood-arterial wall interface. B-scan and other tests measuring alterations in pressure and flow patterns are sensitive only to hemodynamically significant lesions and thus cannot detect smaller plaques or thrombi, which may be responsible for certain embolic phenomena.

Because many strokes, transient ischemic attacks, retinal infarctions, and episodes of amaurosis fugax are attributed to emboli originating from small plaques or ulcerations at the carotid bifurcation, it seemed particularly appropriate to apply the pulsed-Doppler imaging technique to the investigation of extracranial arterial disease. This chapter describes our experience with this modality in a prospective clinical evaluation of patients with suspected carotid arterial disease (4).

INSTRUMENTATION

The Hokanson ultrasonic arteriograph (UA) consists of a 5-MHz pulsed-Doppler flow detector with a 4-mm piezoelectric crystal mounted on the end of a position sensing arm (Fig. 1). Six direction-sensing gates can sample flow simultaneously at six depths along the ultrasonic beam. When a flow signal of the proper direction, frequency, and amplitude is detected, the screen of a storage oscilloscope is activated. Coordinates of the sample volume are determined by the spatial orientation of the probe and by the range information derived from the flow detector.

Two modes of operation are possible. When the probe is aligned with the long axis of the position sensing arm, activation of any or all of the range gates will produce a single dot on the oscilloscope screen. The resulting image is a projection of the artery as seen from the origin of the position sensing arm.

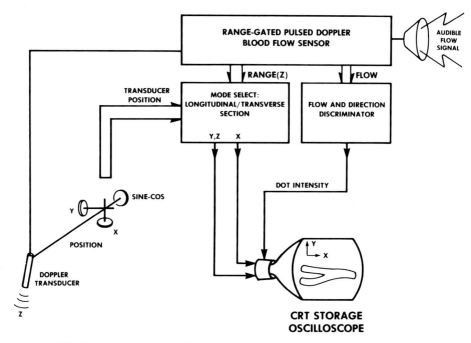

FIG. 1. Components of the Hokanson pulsed-Doppler ultrasonic imaging system.

TABLE 1. *Ability of pulsed-Doppler ultrasonic arteriography
to detect lesions according to degree of stenosis on X-ray*

X-ray % diameter stenosis	Number of vessels	Ultrasonic arteriography % positive studies	
		> 20[a]	> 40[a]
100	18	78	78
80–99	16	94	94
60–79	15	93	93
40–59	20	95	85
20–39	28	61	21
< 19	26	15	15
0	86	12	3

[a]Percent diameter stenosis considered positive.

When the probe is mounted perpendicular to the position sensing arm, a separate dot appears simultaneously on the screen for each gate activated. In this mode, the oscilloscope screen represents the plane in which the ultrasonic beam moves. If the arm is moved across the long axis of the underlying vessel, a transverse cross section is obtained, but if the arm is moved along the long axis of the vessel, a longitudinal cross section appears.

METHODS

To study the cervical carotid artery, the UA probe is aligned with the arm. This provides an image closely resembling a lateral contrast roentgenogram of the carotid bifurcation, with good separation of the internal and external carotids (Fig. 2). After locating the common carotid artery, the operator moves the probe slowly cephalad, carefully interrogating all areas for flow signals, until the internal carotid signal disappears beneath the mandible. Then the external carotid is traced back to

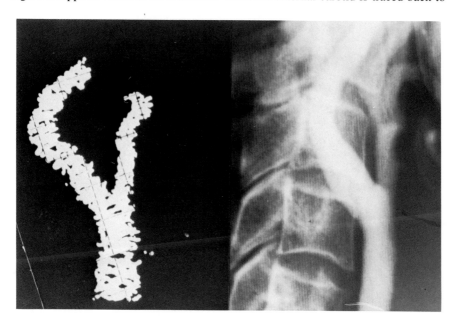

FIG. 2. Ultrasonic arteriogram (**left**) and lateral roentgenogram (**right**) of a normal carotid bifurcation. On each image, the internal carotid artery is on the left and the external carotid is on the right.

TABLE 2. *Ability of pulsed-Doppler ultrasonic arteriography (UA) to discriminate between diameter reductions greater or less than 20%*

	X-ray diameter stenosis	
	< 20%	>20%
UA < 20%	98	18
UA > 20%	14	79
Total	112	97

Specificity = 88% (98/112); sensitivity = 81% (79/97).

TABLE 3. *Ability of pulsed-Doppler ultrasonic arteriography (UA) to discriminate between diameter reductions greater or less than 40%*

	X-ray diameter stenosis	
	< 40%	> 40%
UA < 40%	127	9
UA > 40%	13	60
Total	140	69

Specificity = 91% (127/140); sensitivity = 87% (60/69).

the bifurcation. To avoid artifacts related to movement of the patient, each scan is completed expeditiously (usually within 3 min) without retracing areas previously examined. The audible output of the instrument helps the technician follow the underlying arteries and assess the image.

It is our practice to repeat the scan at least once with the probe at a slightly different angle. If questions still remain, transverse or longitudinal cross sections are obtained. A skilled operator can examine both carotids within 30 min.

MATERIAL

Of 577 patients examined using the UA for suspected extracranial carotid arterial disease, 122 (21%) subsequently underwent X-ray arteriography. Eleven ultrasonic scans (5%) were uninterpretable (only one side was studied in two patients), and unilateral X-rays were obtained in 22 patients. Thus, comparisons were possible between X-ray and UA scans in 209 vessels. In all cases, the UA scan was interpreted prior to obtaining the X-ray.

RESULTS

Typical scans illustrating a stenosis and an occlusion of the internal carotid artery are shown in Figs. 3 and 4, respectively. In the scan and X-ray images, the degree of stenosis was estimated by comparing the diameter of the internal carotid artery at the narrowest point with that of a distal segment of the internal carotid. When the ultrasonic image was difficult to measure (owing to calcification, noise, or other factors), the audible Doppler signal was used to supplement the visual interpretation.

Based on these admittedly crude estimates, near perfect correspondence of the UA and X-ray images was obtained in 131 of 209 (63%) of the studies (Fig. 5). Eighty-four percent of the examinations agreed within 20%.

Table 1 shows the ability of the UA to detect varying degrees of arterial stenosis. Over 90% of all lesions with diameter reductions between 40 and 99% were recognized, and 61% of the low-grade stenoses with diameter reductions between 20 and 40% were detected; however, the false positive incidence was rather high (12%).

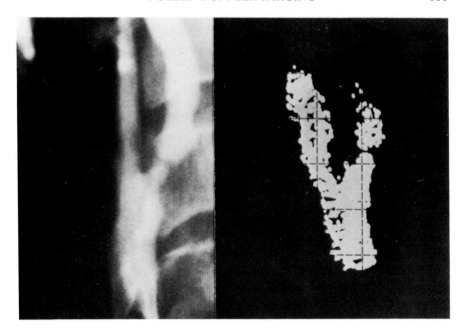

FIG. 3. Stenosis of the internal carotid artery comparison of roentgenogram and ultrasonic arteriogram.

Selecting 40% diameter reduction on the UA as the dividing line decreased the false positive incidence to 3%, but also decreased the ability to detect low-grade stenoses. The apparent rather low sensitivity (78%) of the UA to total occlusion was largely due to misreading of technically satisfactory scans.

Tables 2 and 3 analyze the data in terms of the UA's ability to discriminate between stenoses greater or less than 20% and greater or less than 40%, respectively.

Hemodynamically Insignificant Lesions

Because most noninvasive testing procedures fail to detect small, hemodynamically insignificant lesions, we studied the UA data to determine their accuracy in this regard. As shown in Table 4, most stenoses narrowing the internal carotid by 26 to 50% were recognized, and about half of those between 0 and 25% were detected. There was again, however, a fairly high incidence of false positive studies, with a specificity of only 81%.

Total Versus Near-Total Occlusion

Another shortcoming of the more commonly employed noninvasive tests is their inability to distinguish between severe stenosis and total occlusion of the internal carotid artery. This distinction is of great importance in planning therapy.

The UA was not particularly impressive in this regard (Table 5). In part, this was the result of misinterpreting six technically satisfactory scans showing, in

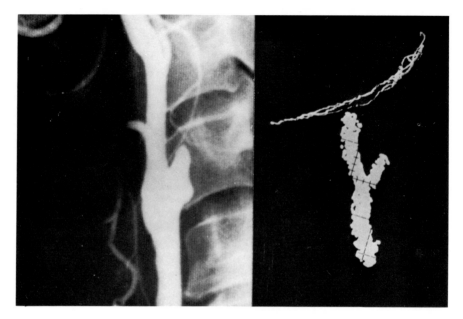

FIG. 4. Occlusion of the internal carotid artery, comparison of roentgenogram and ultrasonic arteriogram.

TABLE 4. *Detection of hemodynamically insignificant lesions by pulsed-Doppler ultrasonic arteriography (UA) (157 vessels)*

	X-ray diameter stenosis		
	0%	≤ 25%	26–50%
UA 0%	(70)	19	3
UA ≤ 25%	8	(10)	5
UA 26–50%	6	5	(20)
UA ≥ 51%	2	3	6
Total	86	37	34

Specificity = 81% (70/86); sensitivity of ≤ 25% group = 49% (18/37); sensitivity of 26–50% group = 91% (31/34); correspondence of figures in parentheses = 64% (100/157).

retrospect, total occlusion of the internal carotid artery. In these views, the external carotid image had been misidentified as the internal. Since these "false negative" studies would have been detected by X-ray prior to any operation, calling a few arteries stenotic, rather than occluded, should not be considered a serious error. On the other hand, if a stenotic artery were misinterpreted as being occluded, an X-ray might not be obtained, and a potentially operable lesion might be missed.

TABLE 5. *Accuracy of pulsed-Doppler ultrasonic arteriography (UA) in distinguishing severe stenosis from total occlusion of the internal carotid artery*

	X-ray diameter stenosis	
	80%–99%	Total occlusion
UA ⩽ 99%	13	8[a]
UA Total occlusion	3	10

[a]Includes six erroneous interpretations of technically satisfactory scans.
Specificity = 81% (13/16); sensitivity = 56% (10/18); sensitivity with proper interpretation of scans = 85% (16/18).

Although the specificity of the UA was fairly good (81%) in the group of patients, missing three of 16 potentially operable lesions is probably not acceptable.

Accuracy According to Presenting Complaint

Because one of the functions of any noninvasive study is to help the clinician decide which patients need arteriography, we examined our results to see how accurately the UA would reflect the patient's presenting complaint (Table 6). Any distinct lesion, regardless of the degree of stenosis, that was detectable on X-ray or UA was considered positive in patients with localizing signs or symptoms (transient ischemic attacks, strokes, amaurosis fugax). In this group, the UA was 89 to 100% sensitive and 80 to 90% specific. A stenosis ⩾ 40% was considered positive in those patients with asymptomatic bruits, since it is likely that operation would not be undertaken in most patients with less severe lesions.

Although the sample was small, the results were encouraging. In patients with nonlocalizing signs or symptoms (syncope, dizziness, diplopia, bilateral visual disturbances, etc.), it is difficult to say what constitutes a significant lesion. With the dividing line between positive and negative studies set at 20%, the UA proved to be fairly sensitive (91%), but the specificity was poor (70%).

SOURCE OF ERRORS

As previously mentioned, most of the false negative errors were due to mistaking the external carotid artery for the internal and identifying the branches of the external carotid artery as the external itself. In retrospect, it was evident that the UA image closely resembled the X-ray image. More experience in interpreting the scans should eliminate these errors. Other causes of false negative studies included failure to follow the internal carotid far enough distally to pick up the stenosis, superimposition of the external and internal carotids, and technical errors.

X-Ray - % Stenosis

Ultrasonic Arteriography - % Stenosis	Neg.	< 20	20 - 40	40 - 60	60 - 80	80 - 100
Neg.	70	15	7	1	1	4
< 20	6	7	4			1
20 - 40	7		11	2		
40 - 60	2	2	6	12	3	5
60 - 80	1	2		5	11	4
80 - 100						20

FIG. 5. Comparison of results of ultrasonic arteriography and X-ray studies of 209 internal carotid arteries from 122 patients. *Crosshatched areas* indicate near perfect correspondence; *stippled areas* represent the most serious errors (4).

TABLE 6. *Accuracy of pulsed-Doppler ultrasonic arteriography (UA) in patients according to presenting complaint*

	Stenosis positive criterion (%)	Number of patients	Sensitivity (%)	Specificity (%)
TIA	> 0	25	93	82
Stroke	> 0	28	89	90
Amaurosis fugax	> 0	13	100	80
Asymptomatic bruit	≥ 40	12	100	100
Nonlocalizing	≥ 20	32	91	70

Most of the false positive results were due to calcification, which results in a sonic opacity that can be misinterpreted as a stenosis or occlusion. In a few cases, the audible signal seemed turbulent; although the image was practically normal, it was deduced that a stenosis was present. Reduced carotid flow due to proximal common carotid disease accounted for a few errors. No cause could be ascertained for the remainder, except inexperience and technical factors.

TABLE 7. *Reported accuracy of ultrasonic arteriography*

Author	Criterion for positive X-ray (%)	Sensitivity (%)	Specificity (%)
Barnes et al. (5)	50	92	65
Wolf (6)	40	93	92
Hobson et al. (7)	50	89	90
Blackshear et al. (8)	50	88	55
Sumner et al. (4)	40	86	90

DISCUSSION

Relatively few reports have documented the accuracy of pulsed-Doppler UA (Table 7). Comparison between these results and those obtained with other non-invasive methods is hampered somewhat by the fact that different investigators tend to employ different criteria for a positive study. Nevertheless, it would appear that the UA has a sensitivity (86 to 93%) comparable to or exceeding that obtainable with other noninvasive tests (4). The reported specificity, however, varies from 55 to 92%; but without examining the raw data, it is difficult to say what these figures mean. A positive scan associated with a stenosis of 30%, for example, would be considered "false positive" when a stenosis of 50% is the chosen dividing line between positive and negative. In fact, the specificity of the UA in the report of Blackshear et al. (8) would increase to 75% if the dividing line were shifted to 10% diameter reduction.

The accuracy of the pulsed-Doppler examination might be improved in several ways. One is by adding another testing modality. In our experience, when the fluid-filled oculoplethysmograph (OPG) and the UA agreed (which they did in 67% of the studies), the sensitivity was 95% and the specificity 94% (4). When they disagreed, unfortunately, one has to choose which test to believe. We found the UA to be the better of the two tests, having a sensitivity of 81% compared with 21% for the OPG. However, a markedly positive OPG test in the presence of an apparently negative scan should encourage one to review the scan, since, in some of these cases, the external carotid will have been misinterpreted as the internal.

The fact that the scan provides an image in only one plane constitutes another problem. It is well known that a stenosis clearly visible on one X-ray may not even be evident on another. Although repeating the scan with the probe at a different angle may eliminate some such errors, this process is time consuming. We have developed a prototype microcomputer system that displays simultaneously two orthogonal images of the carotid bifurcation. Our early experience with this modification has been encouraging.

Finally, one can perform spectral analysis of the Doppler flow signal at selected points along the internal carotid artery, as advocated by Blackshear et al. (8). Supplementing the image with an objective evaluation of the flow signal should reduce the number of errors, particularly when calcification is present.

CONCLUSIONS

Pulsed-Doppler ultrasonic imaging has been demonstrated to be a reasonably accurate method for examining the carotid bifurcation. It is safe, rapid, and well tolerated by the patient. With better interpreter skills, incorporation of flow-signal analysis, computerization of the image, and the possible addition of other noninvasive tests, this technique holds promise for the future.

REFERENCES

1. Mozersky, D. J., Hokanson, D. E., Baker, D. W., Sumner, D. S., and Strandness, D. E., Jr. (1971): Ultrasonic arteriography. *Arch. Surg.*, 103:663.
2. Hokanson, D. E., Mozersky, D. J., Sumner, D. S., McLeod, F. D., Jr., and Strandness, D. E., Jr. (1972): Ultrasonic arteriography, a noninvasive method of arterial visualization. *Radiology*, 102:435.
3. Mozersky, D. J., Hokanson, D. E., Sumner, D. S., and Strandness, D. E., Jr. (1972): Ultrasonic visualization of the arterial lumen. *Surgery*, 72:253.
4. Sumner, D. S., Russell, J. B., Ramsey, D. E., Hajjar, W. M., and Miles, R. D. (1979): Noninvasive diagnosis of extracranial carotid arterial disease. A prospective evaluation of pulsed-Doppler imaging and oculoplethysmography. *Arch. Surg.*, 114:1222.
5. Barnes, R. W., Bone, G. E., Reinertson, J., Slaymaker, E. E., Hokanson, D. E., and Strandness, D. E., Jr. (1976): Noninvasive ultrasonic carotid angiography. Prospective validation by contrast arteriography. *Surgery*, 80:328.
6. Wolf, E. A., Jr. (1979): Discussion of Sumner et al. Noninvasive diagnosis of extracranial carotid arterial disease. *Arch. Surg.*, 114:1229.
7. Hobson, R. W., II, Berry, S. M., O'Donnell, J. A., and Jamil, Z. (1979): Improved accuracy in noninvasive diagnosis of extracranial carotid arterial disease: Combination of pulsed-Doppler ultrasonic imaging (UI) and fluid-filled oculoplethysmography (OPG). *San Diego Symposium on Noninvasive Diagnostic Techniques in Vascular Disease*, p. 35 (*Abstract*).
8. Blackshear, W. M., Jr., Phillips, D. J., Thiele, B. L., Hirsch, J. H., Chikos, P. M., Marinelli, M. R., Ward, K. J., and Strandness, D. E. Jr. (1979): Detection of carotid occlusive disease by ultrasonic imaging and pulsed-Doppler spectrum analysis. *Surgery*, 86:698.

Noninvasive Techniques for Assessment of Atherosclerosis in Peripheral, Carotid, and Coronary Arteries, edited by Thomas F. Budinger, et al. Raven Press, New York 1982.

Ultrasound B-Scan Imaging of Atherosclerosis in Carotid Arteries

Titus C. Evans, Jr.

Cardiovascular Division, Mayo Foundation, Mayo Medical School, Rochester, Minnesota 55901

As a medical cardiologist interested in applied medical research, I have been privileged to participate in the development and testing of ultrasound B-scan arterial imaging equipment with Dr. James Greenleaf and Messrs. William Samayoa and Christopher Hansen of the Mayo Foundation, along with Messrs. Phil Green, Dave Ramsey, John Holzemer, Kenneth Marich, Joseph Suarez and Drs. Jon Taenzer and Peter Edmonds of SRI International Corporation. Our team has been working in this field for seven years, and I am happy to be the spokesman for our group. Other workers, such as Dr. Ralph Barnes and associates at the Bowman Gray School of Medicine, Dr. Charles Olinger and associates at the University of Cincinnati, and Don Baker and associates at the University of Washington, have also done extensive B-scan instrument development and testing for imaging of atherosclerosis.

Two-dimensional echo techniques, which show depth and width, have revolutionized the field of echocardiology. Images from these sector scans actually do look like tomograms of the structures being imaged, as opposed to the older, wavy-lined M-mode scans, which plot depth against time. Two-dimensional arterial B-scans hold the same promise of major advancement in the clinical detection, localization, and quantification of arterial atherosclerotic lesions. The term "B-scan" is used because the brightness of points on the image corresponds to the amount of reflection from acoustical interfaces within the structures being imaged. In arteries containing lesions, the interfaces of blood with arterial walls and lesions, as well as the layers within the lesions, serve as sources of reflection on the B-scan images. Arterial walls and lesions thus appear as bright reflections in contrast to the dark appearance of the blood.

The two-dimensional B-scan display allows the observer to identify the normal position and appearance of the arterial wall and the blood and quickly recognize arterial orientation, size, shape, and position. If real-time displays are employed, actual motion, expansile pulsations, longitudinal translation, and coiling and uncoiling of tortuous arteries are instantly seen. The operator can change the orientation and location of the plane of scanning to achieve the desired images quickly. De-

117

viations from the normal range of findings can be recognized very quickly without delayed computer processing, special image enhancement techniques, development of film, or injection of any form of angiographic or ultrasonic contrast material, such as iodide dye or indocyanine green.

Even more important, atherosclerotic lesions, if large enough and reflective enough, stand out clearly and plainly on the images, so even a novice observer can learn quickly to recognize them. The technique thus has instant appeal to the user and a very direct, practical clinical application in the noninvasive assessment of atherosclerotic lesions. It can determine the presence or absence of lesions, their exact location, and their approximate size and shape. Thus, it allows the operator to estimate the degree of loss of distal blood pressure and flow to the target organ quickly. Lesions can be studied in a large number of planes in several scan directions (usually longitudinal and transverse with respect to the long axis of the artery), and each plane can be scanned at will for as long a time as is required for interpretation. Documentation photographs or videotape images can be made for subsequent inspection and study. Repeat scans can be made during the same imaging session or at any time in the future, allowing serial studies of the growth, regression, alteration of shape, or change in intensity (and thus content) of a given lesion.

Ultrasound B-scanning entails no appreciable penalty, risk, or pain for the person being scanned or for the operator and is essentially a nontraumatizing, minimally invasive method. It involves no photon radiation, iodinated contrast dyes, potential anaphylaxis, potential infection, potential hemorrhage or dissection, potential cerebrovascular accident, pain, discomfort, anesthesiology, etc. and does not require hospitalization or immediate surgical intervention capabilities. Ultrasound B-scans are ideal for screening of atherosclerosis, those at risk for developing it, and those who might be candidates for angiography and arterial surgery.

The inherent features of ultrasound do, however, restrict the usefulness of the B-scan technique. It does not provide all the desirable clinical information, and it has major physical limitations. Doppler flow measurement or other ultrasound techniques are necessary to determine relative streaming patterns and velocity changes as blood flows past, or is prevented from flowing past, an atherosclerotic lesion. A B-scan image of a very highly obstructive lesion (90 to 100% of lumen diameter) does not distinguish completely obstructing lesions from partially obstructing ones. This is critical in the case of carotid artery lesions, as the decision for subsequent angiography and potential corrective artery surgery (endarterectomy) depends largely on this distinction. Given the 2% or greater morbidity risk for carotid angiography and a similar *additional* risk for carotid endarterectomy to remove a lesion, the deficiency of the B-scan in this respect becomes obvious.

In summary, the B-scan can determine quickly and easily whether practically any patient, fat or thin, young or old, with or without a previous cerebrovascular accident or retinal embolus, has carotid artery lesions at the bifurcation or elsewhere within the neck. This technique also reveals where they are located, how large they are (height, width, and approximate shape), and their probable significance in mechanically obstructing flow. (It cannot, however, show actual flow disturbances.)

Our group believes that B-scan and Doppler instruments combined will be the optimum noninvasive clinical ultrasound approach to assessment of atherosclerosis in the carotid arterial system and perhaps in other arteries.

Proper B-scan resolution depends on such criteria as attenuation of all frequencies of ultrasound energy with increasing depth; preferential degradation of the desired high frequencies (which give the best resolution information) with increasing depth; minimal intervening air or bone; and optimal absorption, reflection, and scattering of the intervening and imaged structures themselves. Such superficial structures as the common carotid artery are visualized with slightly higher resolution than deeper structures, like the carotid bulb (where most carotid lesions are found) and, especially, the bifurcation of the internal and external carotid arteries, which lies deep within the neck. Advanced engineering techniques in designing and building the B-scan system and maintenance of ideal physical conditions for our scans allowed our SRI-Mayo team to image carotid artery lesions with relative ease in patients at the Mayo Clinic. We scanned 300 carotid arteries in 150 patients, using a laboratory version of the SRI B-scan system; later, we scanned an identical number of additional arteries and patients, using a more advanced clinical B-scan system. Lesions were seen in many of the 600 arteries scanned, and 60 of these correlated with angiograms. The correlations were generally excellent.

Nonsilhouetted positioning of small carotid lesions and superpositioning of dye before or behind them can make them hard to recognize using conventional radiocontrast angiography. Ultrasound B-scanning, we learned, is distinctly superior in such cases. We found that even highly experienced cerebral radiologists could not reliably see some lesions or significantly underrated them on some of the angiograms. Often, only slight excess in density of the contrast medium concealed their presence. Only close retrospective comparison with the corresponding ultrasound B-scans revealed these lesions.[1]

When we imaged larger lesions using both techniques, the correlation was generally high. The presence or absence of dye distal to a high-grade lesion, seen in the angiogram, gave it an advantage over the ultrasound B-scan in determining completeness of occlusion. At times, especially in very high-grade lesions, the technical limitations of the B-scan technique became apparent. Flow was apparently influenced by additional atherosclerotic disease within the skull beyond the range of the ultrasound scanning system. The lumen sometimes seemed to disappear, and we could not always determine the distal course beyond the lesion, although this was almost exclusively limited to the internal and external carotids. The theoretical resolution of our instrument was 0.6 mm, but we obtained this only at the optimal focal depth of the lens-transducer combination.

One of the most important features of the image of the atherosclerotic lesion on the B-scan is its shadowing of deeper structures, due to overlying reflection or

---

[1] These appeared in patients who later avoided carotid surgery, because the lesions proved small; however, the implications for the two competing techniques are clear.

absorption of much of the ultrasound energy. A bright lesion on the anterior wall often will cast a shadow on the corresponding, or "kissing," portion of the lesion on the posterior wall, darkening its internal structural detail as compared with that of the surrounding atheromata. This may give the false impression that the lesion is bifid or contains an ulcer crater. Differences among various ultrasound instruments may yield differing images, depending on their automatic and manual gain compensation features. If a lesion is very thick in the direction of the ultrasound beam, then a shadow often obstructs the lesion itself. Such shadows may be especially dark under a correspondingly bright (calcified) portion. We are incorporating a gain compensation network in our B-scanner, which will reduce this effect by boosting the strength of the image at the flick of a switch.

Despite the technology to record motion on videotape and make longitudinal and transverse B-scans at multiple arterial levels, it is still difficult to reconstruct mentally the resulting three-dimensional (3-D) image. Clinical acceptance of new techniques requires experience using them, and unfortunately, such experience is often voluntary. Surgical and nonsurgical medical colleagues, who do not use ultrasound routinely, are reluctant to spend the time needed to understand completely or even accept B-scanning of atherosclerotic lesions. Improved 3-D display of the carotid artery in ultrasound scans would greatly help streamline documentation photography sessions and would thus foster more rapid and widespread clinical acceptance.

We mounted the scanning head of our instrument on a flexible, counterbalanced pantograph arm, which permitted the plane of scan to be moved easily or to be held absolutely constant. The scanning transducer and its focusing lens were contained in a flexible, fluid-filled coupling bag. Alpha-Keri bath oil was used to displace air between the patient's skin and the coupling bag; the patient was placed horizontally on an examining table. The shoulder on the side being imaged was elevated 15°, using a pillow, and the patient's head was rotated toward the opposite side an additional 15°, locating the carotid artery at the top of the neck for optimal scanning. The coupling bag was placed gently against the skin of the neck, and the entire scanning head and bag were reoriented when the plane of the scan was changed. The transducer moved back and forth up to 15 times/sec within the coupling bag to provide repeated scans, showing motion in real time.

Pressure of the coupling bag against the neck was limited by a pressure compensation system to not more than 2 cm of water. Since this equals only about 2 or 3 mm of mercury, pressure on the carotid artery by the coupling bag was insignificantly low, with no possibility of compression of the carotid artery. Venous waves in the internal and external jugular veins easily lifted the bag with each cardiac cycle, confirming the innocuous nature of the coupling bag system. Patients tolerated our scans with ease, and a few were so comfortable that they even fell asleep during the scans.

To avoid transient postprocedural orthostatic hypotension, especially important for elderly patients and those with carotid atherosclerosis, we require an important precautionary procedure for all—regardless of age, disease, or scan results: Patients lie still for a full 30 sec after scanning, with the coupling bag off the neck; sit on the edge of the examining table for an additional 30 sec; and, finally, raise their arms over their head while standing up. This maintains the correct heart-filling pressure and prevents faintness.

In summary, we conclude that ultrasound B-scans of the carotid arterial system in the neck are very helpful clinically in their present state of development. Better resolution of lesion detail and reduction of shadowing, however, would allow more precise definition of the structure and perhaps the internal content of lesions. A companion Doppler flow system might supplement this imaging technique to make ultrasound instruments even more useful. Finally, a 3-D display format, usable at, or soon after, the time of the actual scan, would dramatically boost clinical acceptance of ultrasound scans and their usefulness to the clinical physician and the atherosclerosis researcher alike. We are planning these improvements in our own clinical scanning system.

Noninvasive Techniques for Assessment of
Atherosclerosis in Peripheral, Carotid, and
Coronary Arteries, edited by Thomas F.
Budinger, et al. Raven Press, New York
1982.

Duplex Methods in Cardiovascular Disease Detection

Donald W. Baker

Department of Research, Division of Ultrasound, University of Washington,
Seattle, Washington 98105

The duplex approach combines the capabilities of two-dimensional, real-time imaging with blood flow detection and imaging. In its fully expanded form, it can assess tissue properties in relation to local anatomy. It is a holistic approach to increasing the accuracy and sensitivity of plaque diagnosis by combining the capabilities of several modalities in a complementary format.

This approach was spurred by the inherent limitations of existing instruments and shaped by the nature of the atherosclerotic process (1). The use of imaging techniques for plaque detection in peripheral arteries assumes a resolution and sensitivity adequate to detect the pertinent types of plaques. It also assumes an anatomy capable of evaluation by a typical planar imager. Tortuous vessels or other anomalies may render this impossible. This technique further assumes that some form of detectable plaque is always the most significant indication of the diseased state. The experience of many investigators attempting to rely solely on two-dimensional imaging has been less than favorable. Inability to detect soft, acoustically transparent plaques was their primary limitation. (Blood flow alterations cannot be detected using any echo imaging method.)

Any approach based exclusively on blood flow or Doppler techniques will be thwarted by another prohibitive set of limitations. Poor spatial resolution in the blood flow image is a primary problem, as is the excessive time required to carry out the procedure—many cardiac cycles are needed to build up an adequate image. The principal data gained are from the spectral broadening signal caused by flow disturbances due to narrowing or wall roughening. The presence and amount of spectral broadening are extremely sensitive indicators of an anatomical defect. Unfortunately, accurate determination of spectral broadening depends on several instrument parameters as well as knowledge of the measurement site and the position of the sample volume within the vessel of interest.

The combination of a high resolution, real-time imaging system with a multigate pulsed Doppler sensor comes close to overcoming the deficiencies of the individual methods currently being evaluated by many investigators. The ultimate real-time duplex scanner would provide a simultaneous real-time display of blood flow overlying an anatomical image. This would require the development and evaluation of a new transducer array and signal processing technology.

Duplex scanners at the University of Washington feature three different operation and display formats. Each represents one stage of development and is meant for a specific area of application.

PERIPHERAL VASCULAR, PV 1

The PV 1 system uses a three-element, 5-MHz rotor transducer with a pulsed Doppler transducer side arm (2). It is capable of true duplex action, i.e., interactive blood flow detection and production of a two-dimensional, real-time image. It sends approximately 30 images/sec over a 4 × 5 cm field of view. The transducer has a single-sample volume and gets its real-time spectral analysis output from a Honeywell Fast Fourier Transform processor. It has three modes of operation: combined echo-Doppler mode, image-only mode, and Doppler-only mode. The Doppler-only mode is required to attain high pulse repetition rates to overcome aliasing due to high flow velocities. A pediatric version of this system has been used in limited trials in pediatric cardiac applications.

ATL MARK IV DUPLEX SCANNER

The ATL Mark IV Duplex Scanner is made in a 3-MHz cardiac and a 5-MHz peripheral vascular version. It is a commercial form of the PV 1 unit just described, but differs in several important ways from the original system due to manufacturing compromises. Its Mark V scan head uses one of the three rotor transducers for Doppler measurement instead of a separate outrigger Doppler arm. The rotor must be stopped and the appropriate transducer aimed at the vessel of interest in order to measure blood flow. This requires producing a tissue image first, then freezing that image in digital storage; a movable cursor then overlays the reproduced image from memory. The movable cursor indicates the orientation of the Doppler transducer, which can be moved into alignment with the structure of interest in the image, using a servo handle on the scan head. The Doppler output is a time-interval histogram indicating spectral broadening due to flow disturbances at the flow site. This first-generation commercial unit was only recently made available and needs evaluation and optimization to meet the challenges of its intended clinical application.

ECHO MEGA I AND MEGA II

Two advanced developmental systems represent the current state of the art in duplex scanners. The Echo Mega I and Mega II are based on the digital multigate Doppler ideas of Brandestini (3) and the color display systems developed by Eyer (4). They are capable of overlaying flow images on tissue images in both two-dimensional and M-mode displays, in either cardiac or peripheral vascular applications. The tissue images are encoded into a range of colors in gray scale representing echo amplitudes. The magnitude and direction of the flow velocity are mapped into two sets of colors, red for positive velocity and blue for negative velocity. These are overlaid on the tissue image to produce a composite echo-flow map. In cardiac applications, the simultaneous echo-flow image is produced in real time using an M-mode display. In two-dimensional applications, the echo image is frozen in memory, and the flow image is written over it. This methodology, even in its early crude form, yields a staggering increase in information about the combined anatomy and flow site. Its overall impact is yet to be determined. Much development and evaluation remain to be done before we can even begin to assess the superiority of this new approach.

RECOMMENDATIONS FOR THE FUTURE

The combined echo-flow color duplex scanner appears to have more potential for rapid, accurate assessment of carotid artery disorders than any other method. Although complex in design, rapid technological development should speed the evolution of these systems—and at a reasonable cost, considering their apparent effectiveness.

Research and application are needed in many areas to exploit this method. Some of these areas are: Echo-Doppler transducer array development; image processing and display development; microprocessor-based adaptable systems research; studies of fluid dynamics, from basic to applied clinical; Doppler signal analysis and spectral display development; evaluation trials, ranging from basic to clinical.

The full development of echo-Doppler scanners for cardiovascular diagnosis is a big undertaking, requiring a multidisciplinary, integrated team approach in an appropriate medical engineering setting.

Thought must be given to the overall approach, administrative and institutional, as well as medical-technical, needed to carry out this work. Appropriate recognition of these problems by the National Institutes of Health is also mandatory to its successful completion.

REFERENCES

1. Baker, D. W. (1979): A Comprehensive Approach to Cardiac Measurements, *Echocardiology*, edited by C. T. Lancee, pp. 15–27. Martinus NIJHOFF, The Hague.
2. Phillips, D. J., et al. (1979): Carotid artery velocity patterns in normal and stenotic vessels. *Stroke (in press)*.
3. Brandestini, M. A., Eyer, M. K., and Stevenson, J. G. (1979): M/Q mode echocardiography: The synthesis of conventional echo with digital multigate Doppler. In: *Echocardiology*, edited by C. T. Lancee. Martinus NIJHOFF, The Hague.
4. Eyer, M. K., Brandestini, M. A., Phillips, D. J., and Baker, D. W. (1980): Color digital echo/Doppler image presentation. *Ultrasound Med. Biol. (in press)*.

Noninvasive Techniques for Assessment of Atherosclerosis in Peripheral, Carotid, and Coronary Arteries, edited by Thomas F. Budinger, et al. Raven Press, New York 1982.

Cross-Sectional Echocardiographic Visualization of the Coronary Arteries

Arthur E. Weyman

Department of Medicine, Indiana University School of Medicine, University Hospital, Indianapolis, Indiana 46202

Cross-sectional echocardiographic visualization of the left main coronary artery was first described in 1976 (1). This study also noted that areas of left main coronary narrowing and aneurysmal dilatation similar to those seen on angiography may be detected in selected patients. A number of studies have since confirmed the validity of this approach in both the proximal left (2–10) and right (7,8,11) coronary arteries, defined in more detail the echocardiographic anatomy of these vessels (2), evaluated this technique in directly visualizing areas of proximal coronary stenosis (2–6,10), explored more sophisticated methods for processing reflected ultrasonic signals in lesion detection (5), and described the echocardiographic features of other anatomic deformities, such as multiple coronary artery aneurysms (7,8) and anomalous origins of both the left and right coronary systems (9).

The frequency with which various segments of the coronary arteries have been visualized echocardiographically is summarized in Table 1. The left coronary ostium has been successfully recorded in from 90 to 99% of adult patients with coronary artery disease (5,10) and in nearly all such pediatric patients (9). The left main coronary segment has been slightly more difficult to visualize, the success rates

TABLE 1. *Reported success rates in imaging various segments of the coronary system*

Ref.	Number patients	LCA Ostium	LMCA	Bifurcation/ LAD	Circulatory	PRCA
Ogawa et al. (3)	35	—	27 (77%)	—	12 (34%)	—
Chen et al. (4)	32	—	—	17 (59%)	—	—
Rogers et al. (5)	100	90 (90%)	—	—	—	—
Friedman et al. (6)	53	—	42 (79%)	—	—	—
Yoshikawa et al. (7)	37	37 (100%)	29 (78%)	—	—	17 (46%)
Aronow et al. (10)	93	—	54 (58%)	—	—	—
Rink et al. (11)	72	71 (99%)	71 (99%)	—	—	—
Total	422	198 (96%)	223 (78%)	17 (59%)	12 (34%)	17 (46%)

varying between 58 and 99% of adult patients (mean, 78%). The bifurcation has been detected in 62% of normal persons and 57% of patients with coronary obstruction (4). The circumflex branch is the most difficult of the left-sided vessels to record; in one study, it was visualized in only 34% of the cases (3). The right coronary artery is uniformly more difficult to visualize than the left. The right coronary success rate has been recorded for one study only, for which it was 46% (7).

The detection of stenotic lesions of the proximal coronary system has been the subject of major research. Atherosclerosis is by far the most common cause of coronary artery stenosis, with atherosclerotic involvement most frequently seen in the proximal segments of these vessels. This predominantly proximal locus is accessible, fortunately, to echocardiographic imaging.

Two characteristic features of atherosclerotic coronary lesions that correspond to the pathologic nature of the disorder have been echocardiographically described. The first is marked by increased echoing from either anterior or posterior margins of the vessel along with loss of the normal parallel echo orientation and reduction or disappearance of the continuous, echo-free space characteristic of the vascular lumen. This pattern is thought to follow the encroachment of the atherosclerotic process on the arterial lumen. The second feature is an abnormal increase in echo intensity at specific points along the vessel, presumably representing areas of increased reflectivity of the vascular walls in an atherosclerotic region, with or without associated vascular narrowing.

The sensitivity and specificity of these criteria for detecting coronary lesions are difficult to assess. Although many studies have addressed these questions, each has utilized different instrumentation, examining techniques, diagnostic criteria for coronary lesions, or methods of image processing. Despite these limitations, there is enough consistency in the results to suggest some general patterns.

Table 2 summarizes available data on the sensitivity and specificity of the cross-sectional technique in directly visualizing left main coronary lesions. Since these

TABLE 2. *Standard echo*

LMCA		+	−	
Angiography	+	33	8	41
	−	38	154	172
		51	162	

Sensitivity	$\dfrac{33}{41}$	= 80%
Specificity	$\dfrac{154}{172}$	= 89%
Pred. V.	$\dfrac{33}{51}$	= 64%

numbers are from a small group of preliminary reports, they merely reflect general trends and cannot in themselves be considered significant. They do suggest, however, that left main coronary lesions can be detected in most cases. False negatives were reported in only one study (6), while false positives occurred fairly often.

Despite these encouraging results, the coronary arteries remain notoriously difficult to record, due to their resolution limitations, the continuous movement of the vessels in and out of the examining plane, and variations in normal coronary anatomy. Several signal processing techniques, however, can help overcome these difficulties. One of these amplificatioin circuits is described in Fig. 1. In this format, the raw low-intensity echoes entering the system (panel A) are logarithmically amplified, which increases their intensity to a detectable level and compresses them into a uniform image field of gray. The midrange echoes (panel B) are linearly amplified and displayed over three shades of gray, as indicated on the output scale. The high-intensity echoes may then be variably amplified using one of a series of formats, from logarithmic to exponential. Panel C shows an exponential amplifi-

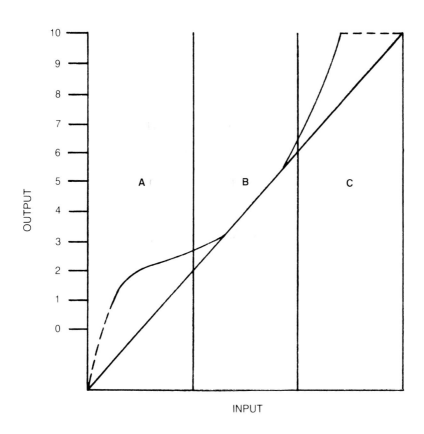

FIG. 1. An echo amplification pattern.

TABLE 3. *Antilog echo*

LMCA		+	−	
Angiography	+	27	0	27
	−	54	63	117
		81	63	

Sensitivity	$\dfrac{27}{27}$	= 100%
Specificity	$\dfrac{63}{117}$	= 54%
Pred. V.	$\dfrac{27}{81}$	= 33%

cation format, which markedly increases the amplitide of the higher intensity echoes and displays them over the final four shades of gray. This format tends to accentuate the higher intensity reflected signals and present them in sharp contrast to the more uniform, logarithmically compressed lower amplitude reflections. In preliminary clinical studies using this type of signal processing, areas of increased reflectivity or echoes of higher intensity were noted in the region of the proximal coronary arteries in patients with atherosclerotic disease.

Table 3 illustrates the sensitivity and specificity of this form of image processing in detecting atherosclerotic lesions in the left main artery, combining the results of two studies. In each of 27 patients having significant stenosis of the left main coronary artery, high-intensity echoes were evident on the cross-sectional scan; further, there were no patients with left main coronary lesions in whom these high-intensity echoes were not produced. Fifty-four patients producing high-intensity echoes, however, did not have left main coronary lesions, but most had lesions elsewhere in the proximal coronary system. This suggests that although high-intensity reflections cannot be considered specific for left main coronary obstruction, they are a highly sensitive indicator of left main coronary lesions.

Available data thus indicate that while the cross-sectional technique cannot specifically detect lesions in the proximal coronary arteries, coronary visualization in a small group of patients, using standard imaging processing methods combined with variable function processing, has proved highly sensitive. This suggests that even though direct visualization of stenotic lesions may not prove possible, cross-sectional exclusion of the presence of obstructing lesions in the left main coronary artery alone may yet be of great clinical value. Although this technology is embryonic and progress has been slow, its potential is great, and it is clearly worthy of continued effort and interest.

REFERENCES

1. Weyman, A. E., Feigenbaum, H., Dillon, J. C., Johnston, K. W., and Eggleton, R. C. (1976): Noninvasive visualization of the left main coronary artery by cross-sectional echocardiography. *Circulation*, 54:169.

2. Rogers, E. W., Feigenbaum, H., Weyman, A. E., Godley, R. W., Wills, E. R., and Vakili, S. T. (1979): Evaluation of coronary artery anatomy *in vitro* by cross-sectional echocardiography. *Am. J. Cardiol.*, 43:386.

3. Ogawa, S., Hubbard, F. E., Pauletto, F. J., Chaudry, K. R., Chen, C. C., Moghadam, A. N., and Dreifus, L. S. (1978): A new approach to noninvasive left coronary artery visualization using phased array cross-sectional echocardiography. *Circulation II*, 58:729.

4. Chen, C. C., Morganroth, J., Mardelli, T. J., Ogawa, S., and Meicell, L. L. (1979): Differential density and luminal irregularities as criteria to detect disease in the left main coronary artery by apex phased array cross-sectional echocardiography. *Am. J. Cardiol.*, 43:386.

5. Rogers, E. W., Feigenbaum, H., Weyman, A. E., Dillon, J. C., Wann, L. S., Eggleton, R. C., and Johnston, K. W. (1978): Possible detection of coronary atherosclerosis by cross-sectional echocardiography. *Circulation II*, 58:209.

6. Friedman, M. J., Sahn, D. J., Goldman, S., Eisner, D. R., Gittinger, N. C., Lederman, F. L., Puckette, C. M., and Tiemann, J. J. (1979): High frequency, high resolution cross-sectional (2D) echo for evaluation of left main coronary artery disease (LMCAD): Is resolution alone enough? *Circulation II*, 60:596.

7. Yoshikawa, J., Yanagihara, K., Owaki, T., Kato, H., Takagi, Y., Okumachi, F., Fukaya, T., Tomita, Y., and Baba, K. (1979): Cross-sectional echocardiographic diagnosis of coronary artery aneurysms in patients with the mucocutaneous lymph node syndrome. *Circulation*, 59:133.

8. Hiraishi, S., Yashiro, K., and Kusano, S. (1979): Noninvasive visualization of coronary arterial aneurysm in infants and young children with mucocutaneous lymph node syndrome with two-dimensional echocardiography. *Am. J. Cardiol.*, 43:1225–1233.

9. Caldwell, R. L., Weyman, A. E., Girod, D. A., Hurwitz, R. A., and Feigenbaum, H. (1978): Cross-sectional echocardiographic differentiation of anomalous left coronary artery from primary myocardiopathy. *Circulation II*, 58:786.

10. Aronow, W. S., Chandraratna, P. A. N., Murdock, K., and Milholland, H. (1979): Left main coronary artery patency assessed by cross-sectional echocardiography and coronary arteriography. *Circulation II*, 60:565.

11. Rink, L. D., Feigenbaum, H., Marshall, J. E., Godley, T. W., Doty, D., Dillon, J. C., and Weyman, A. E. (1980): Improved echocardiographic technique for examining the left main coronary artery. Presented at the *29th Annual Scientific Session of the American College of Cardiology*, Houston, Texas, March 9–13.

12. Yoshikawa, J., Owaki, T., Kato, H., Yanagihara, K., Takagi, Y., and Okumachi, F. (1978): Ultrasonic features of anomalous origin of the left coronary artery from the pulmonary artery. *Jpn. Heart J.*, 19:46.

Noninvasive Techniques for Assessment of Atherosclerosis in Peripheral, Carotid, and Coronary Arteries, edited by Thomas F. Budinger, et al. Raven Press, New York 1982.

Commentary

Peter N. T. Wells

Department of Medical Physics, Bristol General Hospital, Bristol, United Kingdom

I will comment, from a physicist's point of view, on the previous chapters, beginning with the chapter by Drs. Reid and Spencer. Dr. Reid wrote that he thinks his technique of ultrasonic imaging, using the Doppler effect, has eliminated the need for angiography in clinical practice, except as a preliminary to surgery.

It seems to me a tremendously important claim that patients who are going to require some kind of clinical care or are a cause for clinical concern may benefit from the technique of Doppler imaging. This procedure would allow doctors to postpone angiography until such patients reach a stage when they are almost certainly going to need surgery. That would be a tremendous advance, but I see quite a number of difficulties.

Ultrasound is extremely economical, but it is not very good for assessing generalized narrowing, nor is angiography. One of the big drawbacks in the use of both pulsed and continuous-wave Doppler ultrasound is the shadows it produces, particularly around calcified lesions.

There does not seem to be a satisfactory explanation of what causes the shadowing. Some say that it is due to calcium in the lesion, and very likely that is one of the mechanisms. I will return to that theory again when I discuss what the future holds and what we may do to avoid some of these difficulties.

Significantly, both Dr. Reid and Dr. Spencer extract information from ultrasound signals that does not appear on the displays. They depend on their operators or on their own skill in picking out such information from the signals.

This is quite common in many other applications of ultrasound. The question of conveying the information in a permanent record in a way that does not vary with operator skill arises in several areas, particularly in Doppler ultrasound. Furthermore, it is going to be very difficult for Doppler ultrasonic techniques to be accepted by the general clinical community without the development of easily understood methods of displaying the information and of analyzing it.

Dr. Reid mentioned that he finds ultrasound images very useful for picking out regions from which to extract wave forms for subsequent analysis. The matter of wave form analysis has received only a little attention here; we have to look to the future to see what extra information we could get from it.

The mystery of the inverted signals, as mentioned by Drs. Reid and Spencer, is fascinating. I am sure that they do not think that we should all accept their explanation without question. I think that they are not particularly happy with the explanation, but it is most intriguing from the physics and hemodynamic points of view and certainly deserves to be investigated as soon as possible.

Now I will turn to Dr. Sumner's chapter *(this volume)* in which he mentioned conventional B-scanning. He wrote that the echoes do not reliably define the blood/arterial wall interface.

In his chapter, he mentioned a very important point: access to the cranium is impossible when simply looking at the carotids. It is not possible to go very high up in the carotid arteries. For example, one might think that there was a complete blockage when, in fact, a little farther up one would find flow beyond the stenosis.

Dr. Sumner uses pulsed Doppler equipment, and the pictures he used were in the same projection as images made by continuous-wave Doppler instruments. He mentioned that a new projection system being developed should be extremely useful.

I wonder why, if the lumens really are circular, as we have read, a pulsed Doppler system is needed. The problem of shadowing and disappearance of the lumen in particular sections ought not to occur in a circular field. We ought to be able to see the circular lumen using a continuous-wave Doppler system.

The pulsed Doppler system has a number of drawbacks. It is much more elaborate, from an instrumentation point of view. If the continuous-wave systems really do as well, more people might use Doppler.

Now let me turn to Dr. Evans' chapter *(this volume)*. He began by writing about the advantages of real-time ultrasound, and I think they cannot be overemphasized. When looking at the real-time images, one can see how the structures pulse and move relative to each other. It is remarkable that very slow imaging systems that depend on hand scanning, like the continuous-wave Doppler imaging system, produce such good pictures.

It appears that the pulsation of the vessel is predominantly deeper and superficial, rather than from side to side. That may be one of the reasons why the continuous-wave Doppler images are so satisfactory, although the vessel is pulsating in depth rather than laterally. It would be hard to imagine that the continuous-wave Doppler system would be satisfactory if it were pulsating laterally. In slow pulsed Doppler imaging systems, that pulsation must certainly degrade the picture, perhaps much more than we had previously expected.

In a later chapter, Dr. Greenleaf *(this volume)* describes the work involving three-dimensional display at the Mayo Clinic, which is certainly one of the ways that Doppler imaging and pulse echo imaging could be made more acceptable to clinicians.

Dr. Evans *(this volume)* mentioned that a companion Doppler system is expected to be enormously useful. Dr. Baker *(this volume)* presented beautifully the advantages of having a companion Doppler system.

By this ingenious method of display, combining color coding with the structural information obtained from the B-scan, it is possible to see the flow patterns and abnormalities in them. Those techniques should be acceptable to clinicians. They are easily understood, and I think that many surgeons will soon expect and demand this kind of accessory.

Dr. Weyman (*this volume*) has shown us some pictures of the coronary arteries. I was impressed by the remarkable degree of structure recognition in the pictures, which were quite stable, until he showed some gray-scale pictures. Perhaps he will tell us how often it is possible to get such clear definition and resolution of the tiny blood vessels in the myocardium. He displayed a table showing the percentage of patients in which the structures were recognized, but I suspect that the addition of some kind of ultrasonic contrast medium, as was necessary in the early days of echocardiography, might give the rest of us more confidence in the usefulness of that percentage.

He also wrote about tissue characterization and measuring the effects on the myocardium of occlusions in the coronary arteries. This is very interesting and perhaps one of the most likely ways of getting useful information from ultrasound assessment of the coronary arteries, which are extremely difficult to study. The heart is a moving structure with a very limited access through the chest wall. It is an extremely formidable problem to visualize the coronary artery satisfactorily.

It is relatively easy to look at the peripheral arteries (the arteries in the leg), but we have heard no discussion of them. The pulsed and continuous-wave Doppler imaging systems and the new real-time scanners that can image the arteries in the leg have an enormous role to play in the clinical care of patients with vascular disease. These systems could become even more useful with some extra development.

Dr. Schwartz (*this volume*) pointed out the need for high resolution, and Dr. Evans and others wrote about prospects for high-resolution ultrasonic imaging.

Dr. Glagov (*this volume*) pointed out that neither angiography nor, by implication, Doppler ultrasound can show generalized narrowing. Perhaps pulsed echo imaging *can* show generalized narrowing when combined with tissue characterization or some sort of echo discrimination technique.

Transient ischemic attacks are always an emergency and, as Dr. Toole (*this volume*) pointed out, ultrasound is a tremendously useful, noninvasive, very rapid method for dealing with this emergency.

It was pointed out that noninvasive testing is needed, rather than invasive, to establish pre- and postoperative hemodynamic status. Noninvasive testing, particularly ultrasonic imaging and ultrasonic measurement, gives information about function and hemodynamics that we cannot obtain in other ways.

Dr. Budinger (*personal communication*) thought that the single-element imaging systems are the preferred design, and I agree with him at the moment, although serious problems remain to be solved in using ultrasonic arrays. We can expect single-element systems to point the direction in which solid state and switched arrays ought to be developed in order to make these machines inexpensive, reliable, and easy to use.

I found Dr. Carson's chapter (*this volume*) most interesting from the point of view of quality control and the development of phantoms. He emphasized the importance of quality control and proper performance specifications in keeping the reliability of ultrasonic imaging equipment as high as possible.

Finally, Dr. Budinger's recommendation on tissue characterization was brought up several times in discussion of myocardial imaging and clots.

What are the new directions for ultrasound, particularly relative to the goals of this volume?

I want to pick out four or five points. First, there is the matter of risk. It seems to me that this is one question about which we need not be too concerned. There is no evidence that ultrasound is damaging. Occasionally, we see cautionary papers in the literature—for example, one recently in *Radiology* and republished in *Science*—reporting DNA transformations due to diagnostic ultrasound levels. These things occur from time to time, but whether we should be worried about risks depends on the clinical state we are examining. If you are looking at a patient who has a large or dangerous clot, then the potential of long-term damage to that artery due to a marginally possible ultrasonic effect is one that I think ought not to concern us too much. Dr. Barber's point about the danger of probes pushing and shoving on the blood vessels is more relevant and one to consider carefully.

From the technical point of view, the further development of ultrasonic imaging techniques presents a few points to consider. Real-time or rapid Doppler imaging techniques were mentioned as a possibility by Dr. Reid. Anyone who has used a continuous-wave or pulsed Doppler imaging system will know how tedious and lengthy their scanning procedures are. Real-time equipment, at least the rapid Doppler imaging version, is going to be tremendously helpful, particularly considering the pulsations of the blood vessels.

The phenomenon of shadowing by plaques is one from which a lot of information is extracted. Clinicians infer the presence of plaques from a specific type of shadow. Unfortunately, this can give rise to errors and artifacts. A colleague of mine, Dr. Woodcock of Bristol, suggested that echoes from the blood within the vessel might be used as a biological reflection standard for measuring the loss of ultrasound signal strength as it travels to the vessel lumen and back. Compensation could then be made for attentuation in the intervening tissues, particularly in clots.

There has been no discussion of the measurement of inelasticity of blood vessels. Researchers are, in fact, measuring the extensibility of the blood vessel and the thickness of the wall using ultrasonic methods and, from that, are calculating Young's modulus for the arterial wall, for example. Guiding the ultrasonic beam for extracting signals in waveform analysis is a technique that, I think, has a big future. The study of waveforms in some of the more advanced laboratories extends beyond the stage discussed by Dr. Barnes *(this volume)*. Waveforms are being analyzed to extract information about the elasticity and degree of vasodilation or vasoconstriction of the periphery and the proximal lumen diameter of the vessel, based on certain types of modeling. By mathematically matching the waveforms to a simple equation, it is possible to extract information in simple cases.

Finally, degree of resolution is a very important problem. I have noted the very low frequency being used at present—up to 10 MHz. It might be possible to use an extremely high frequency, perhaps 100 MHz, to make very highly detailed images of clots. The pulsation of the clot seems to be quite reproducible and might be measurable using a high- and low-frequency imaging system. Acoustic microscopy might then be adapted to the *in vitro* situation to determine the structure of the plaque. High frequency systems require placement of the transducer near the tissue of interest, thus somewhat invasive vascular probes are required.

Noninvasive Techniques for Assessment of
Atherosclerosis in Peripheral, Carotid, and
Coronary Arteries, edited by Thomas F.
Budinger, et al. Raven Press, New York
1982.

Commentary

William H. Oldendorf

*Department of Neurology, School of Medicine, University of California at Los Angeles,
Los Angeles, California 90024*

I want to make a number of separate comments. I would like to outline a possible application of continuous-wave Doppler that has not, to my knowledge, been exploited. I wrote about this in 1962 (2).

The peculiar location of the middle cerebral artery in the human should allow its use in continuous velocity monitoring. The internal carotid comes up on the left and becomes the middle cerebral artery, running laterally. The right side does the opposite.

First, aim a broad beam of ultrasound into the head laterally, through the temporal bone, at about the position we used to use for midline displacement of the third ventricle. Then look at the backscattered Doppler coming from this cone of tissue. There are two reasons why the blood seen in the ventral cerebral artery will be the source of maximal Doppler shift.

First, the velocity of blood in the middle cerebral artery is the highest in any of the major cerebral vessels.

The middle cerebral artery bifurcates to supply approximately the entire aspect of cerebral hemisphere that is seen from the side. As each artery bifurcates, the combined area of the two branches increases by about a fourth, and the velocity drops by about a fourth, from about a meter/sec in the aortic arch to about a mm/sec in the capillary. The larger the vessel, the greater the velocity.

The middle cerebral arteries pass laterally, the left artery going to the left hemisphere of the brain and the right to the right hemisphere. The flow within this vessel should cause the greatest Doppler shift, because it has the highest velocity and also because of the cosine function of the Doppler shift, that is, the Doppler shift is the cosine of the angle made with the beam times the fraction of the velocity of propagation times the frequency.

The fact that these arteries are in line with the direction of observation would make that cosine factor equal to 1. That maximizes the frequency shift that the middle cerebral artery should produce. Therefore, if one were to observe the frequency shifts from the left side (from the left middle cerebral artery), one would get a shift upward in frequency and a shift downward from the right middle cerebral artery.

The maximal frequency displacement should be obtained from these signals coming from within the head and should represent the flow in the middle cerebral artery. Since this is pulsatile, it will vary.

One might design circuitry to record only the extremes of Doppler shift and to display them as a running number. For a patient in an intensive care unit, for example, mean velocity in the right and left middle cerebral artery might be displayed continuously, which would tell the attendant the status of flow in these two hemispheres. Its major application would be in intensive care, where ordinarily, one is most interested in the integrity of cerebral flow to the middle of the hemisphere.

I have seen images from several scanning systems designed to show the carotid, between the clavicle and the angle of the mandible, in great detail. They are spectacular pictures.

Keep in mind that I am talking about a very restricted view of the great vessel tree in a small region of the neck. In the area of the left common and the left subclavian and the right common and right subclavian arteries, there are many other bifurcations, important potential sites of atherosclerosis, which could cause trouble in the brain if restricted.

Unfortunately, this little segment of carotid artery is the only available site that we may image with good detail and reproducibility. Given this limitation, it is possible to make an angiogram of this area without significant injury to the patient.

In 1958, in *Neurology* (1), I described 80 potential internal carotid artery occlusions that had been assessed using what I call a small-dose angiogram. Using a sharp 20- or 21-gauge needle on a 2½ ml glass-barreled syringe, you can get a much higher pressure at a given thumb force than by using a larger syringe, because of the smaller cross-sectional area of the piston.

A small syringe allows you to inject a substantially greater amount of the viscous contrast medium. The smaller the needle, the less trauma inflicted on the artery. Furthermore, in order to insert a needle big enough for a standard clinical angiogram by direct carotid puncture, you must first collapse the artery. The two walls then come into apposition, and it becomes difficult to maneuver a large needle in between them. But with a 20- or 21-gauge needle, arterial puncture becomes very simple. The artery is readily punctured without collapsing. Using subtraction techniques, one could even use a 21- or 22-gauge needle and perhaps 0.5 cc of dye. This would involve a lot less trauma to the vessel and a lot less osmotic shock to the brain. Trauma to the artery is a function of the length of time it is invaded—a fact not often discussed. The longer an invasive element remains in an artery, the more the vessel relaxes to accommodate the intruder. The longer the needle is left in, the more residual reaction and bleeding will occur when it is pulled out.

In our work, my collaborators and I used a 3 mm copper cone as a shield, exposing only the carotid system and the center of the hemisphere. The puncture was made in about 1 sec, then the dye was injected and the exposure made. This gives an excellent visualization of the carotid bifurcation.

So I suggest that there are better means by which one could look at this restricted area.

Another concern of mine is the lack of interest in actual imaging of the brain using ultrasound. This is largely due to the empirical observation that, after about 2 or 3 years of age, patients no longer yield a significantly distinct ultrasound image of the brain.

The reason for this loss of useful brain image is probably the development of the skull trabecular spaces. Prior to 2 to 4 years of age, the skull is unilaminar. This unilaminar bone structure allows very good ultrasound penetration.

When the skull becomes trabeculated, with an outer table of dense bone, an inner table of dense bone, and the trabeculated space in between, its numerous irregular water-bone interfaces make the skull effectively opaque to ultrasound. The hair is opaque as well and is a major scattering medium.

There is one exception to this, which I think should be exploited. There is an area in the skull (a portion of the temporal bone that covers a part of the temporal lobe) that has no water-bone spaces in the adult. It is quite flat; it remains unilaminar, as in the infant. There are points on this area at which one could scan the head with ultrasound. Sector scans have been made there from a focal point outside the head.

If one were to design a system in which the focal point lay within the body, in this case within part of the temporal bone, it might also be of use in the chest and elsewhere.

In view of the galloping growth rate of technology, CT scanning will probably not be used after another 5 to 10 years. Indeed, part of my reason for not trying in 1964 to interest industry in developing CT was that I felt that ultrasound was going to replace it.

My final point has to do with tissue characterization.

When ultrasound interacts with tissue, one of three things will happen to it: It will be dissipated locally as heat, it will be reflected in a specular fashion if the body with which it is interacting is large, or a part of the energy will be backscattered.

When you change from an object that is large in relation to the wavelength of the ultrasound to an object that is substantially smaller than the wavelength, there is a shift from specular reflection to backscatter.

Specular reflection obeys reflectance laws; that is, the angle of incidence equals the angle of reflection. In backscattering, the emission is isotropic: The rays go equally in all directions. This is a frequency- or wavelength-independent phenomenon. Specular reflection is not isotropic and is frequency independent.

Backscatter follows the Rayleigh fourth power law. This tells us that the amount of backscattering is strongly a function of the ultrasound frequency.

The early scanners used a bimodal display, which showed occasional tall spikes in the return from the tissues. We called this "grass." The grass was clipped off, and the spikes were displayed at a given intensity.

In the early seventies, the bimodal display was discarded in favor of presentation of the entire returned signal, but with attenuation of the gain for the high signals, which were effectively clipped off.

When using specular reflection only, you have to surround the object completely in order to fill in the entire periphery of whatever you are looking at. With backscattering, that is not necessary. You need not look at it from any particular direction, because scattering is isotropic.

We should try to produce an ultrasound picture of the body by assigning a number to each region of the parenchyma of an organ as we do in CT scanning. In the case of an uncontrasted CT scan, this would be almost directly proportional to the organ's regional specific gravity. This would obviate the need to consider regional interfaces.

An important tissue characteristic to display as a number is its scattering cross section or some other characteristic directly related to scattering.

We need to develop a series or class of instruments that can accept both mixed scattering and specular reflection, processing specular reflection in one way and scattering in another, and recombine them in some meaningful way in the final display.

Hopefully, this would give us a picture that more closely resembles that produced by the X-ray CT scan.

The reason scattering is of such interest in tissue characterization is that the degree of scattering of the given tissue varies according to the tissue element doing the scattering.

At 1.5 MHz, ultrasound exhibits a wavelength in water of 1 mm. At 5 MHz, it will be about 0.3 mm. At 5 MHz, objects larger than about 1 μm will become much more effective scatterers by the fourth power function as they increase in size toward 300 μm.

We do not know which elements in tissue are doing the scattering—perhaps collagen fibers, acting like little dipoles are a source. I suspect that mitochondria are especially effective as scatterers.

Mitochondria are stiff structures. They are double-walled on the outside, and they have a whole set of cristi as cross-structures. They make up about 25 to 30% of the liver, for example, and a large fraction of most tissues.

There are many elements in tissue, having various acoustical properties. The great variety of scattering structures exhibit a richness of dimensional and mechanical properties that, as Dr. Weyman *(this volume)* pointed out, should allow frequency analysis of backscattering using the Rayleigh fourth power function and allow characterization of tissue well beyond what we have seen to date.

REFERENCES

1. Oldendorf, W. H. (1958): Demonstration of carotid occlusion by small dose arteriography. *Neurology*, 8:296–298.
2. Oldendorf, W. H. (1962): Speculations on the instrumentation of the nervous system. *Proceedings San Diego Symposium for Biomedical Engineering*, 2:274–280.

*Noninvasive Techniques for Assessment of
Atherosclerosis in Peripheral, Carotid, and
Coronary Arteries*, edited by Thomas F.
Budinger, et al. Raven Press, New York
1982.

Tomography of Hydrogen by Nuclear Magnetic Resonance: A New Way to Detect Atherosclerosis?

Lawrence Crooks, John Hoenninger, Mitsuaki Arakawa,
Leon Kaufman, Robert McRee, Jeffrey Watts, Robert Herfkens

*Radiologic Imaging Laboratory, University of California,
South San Francisco, California 94080*

Nuclear magnetic resonance (NMR) imaging is a noninvasive technique that can map hydrogen distributions in intact animals. It has attracted a great deal of attention because it is apparently nonhazardous and because the intrinsic NMR contrast ratio is higher than that of X-ray contrast. On the other hand, the *in vivo* NMR characteristics of normal and abnormal tissues are not well understood and are just beginning to be studied.

The basic principle of NMR is that all nuclei with an odd number of protons or neutrons behave like small magnets. Placed in an external magnetic field, they will align their magnetic moment with that of the field. The magnetic moment can be flipped or turned around using radio waves of a specific energy level. This energy level or frequency is related to the magnetic field at the nucleus, H_{Loc}, as:

$$f = \gamma \, H_{Loc}$$

where γ is a constant representing the gyromagnetic ratio of the particular type of nucleus. As it returns to the normal state, a flipped nucleus will either radiate back these radio waves or dissipate its energy thermally by coupling it to paramagnetic atoms in the surrounding material.

This property allows one to assess the NMR absorption spectrum of an object by observing the energy emitted by its nuclei in response to a low-level radio frequency pulse. Upon placement of a specimen in a position-variant (having an intensity that varies with its position) magnetic field, the frequencies of nuclei at different positions will vary accordingly. A frequency discriminant is thus provided for nuclei at differing positions, with the nuclear density of a unit or element of volume within an excited volume of atoms represented by the intensity of a particular frequency of the NMR signal.

A planar volume of nuclei in the sample can be excited by exposing the sample to a magnetic field variation and a radio wave in such a way that only the desired

143

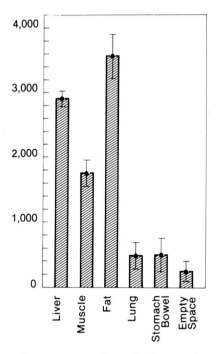

FIG. 1. Signal intensities for various tissues in the live rat show a large range of values, indicative of the high intrinsic contrast found in NMR imaging.

plane corresponds to the frequencies of the radio wave. By varying the direction of the field, two intersecting planes can be excited. A signal known as a spin echo will later be emitted by only the nuclei along the line of intersection of the two excited planes. The spin echo thus contains information about only those nuclei. By applying a field variation along this line, frequency discrimination of the emitted radio waves is produced along the line. A tomographic image is then built up by moving the line through the desired plane. The NMR intensity is proportional to the nuclear density, but may be modified by two nuclear magnetization decay rates, known as T_1 and T_2. Areas with a long T_1 (> 1.0 sec) will have reduced intensity, and areas with a short T_2 (< 0.1 sec) will have reduced intensity. Since hydrogen is the molecule with the most abundant odd mass-number nucleus among animals, NMR is ideally suited for mapping its density (which differs significantly from electron density as measured by computerized tomography or other X-ray techniques).

Our NMR imager uses a Varian magnet with a 30-cm gap, operated at 0.352 T (15 MHz hydrogen-resonant frequency). The imager can accept a cylindrical object up to 6.5 cm in diameter. The measured resolution (1) is 0.5×2.0 mm² full width (FW) in the image plane with a slice thickness of 8.4 mm.

For an image 24 lines high (4.8 cm high, 6.4 cm wide), the contrast resolution achieved in an imaging time of 5 min is 3.5%. Figure 1 shows the relative image intensities of various tissues in a live rat. Figure 2 shows six images of various sections of a live rat, with high signal intensities shown as bright regions.

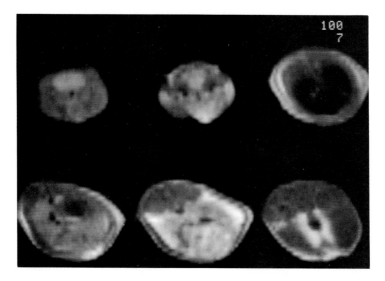

FIG. 2. Six sections through a rat, each done in 5 min. **Upper left** and **middle** images are from the head. Visible are the brain (**top**), eyes, and surrounding bone (low intensity). **Upper right** image is the chest with the air-filled lungs showing as dark areas. **Lower sections** are through the abdomen. The **middle image** shows the back muscle on the upper left and the spine as a dim spot. **Right image** shows the rectum.

There are two ways in which NMR could help detect atherosclerotic plaques. One is measurement of blood flow, and the other is imaging of plaque in large vessels.

NMR has measured velocity distribution *in vivo* (2). Although giving no spatial resolution, it should be possible to limit this type of measurement at least to a planar region. Our imaging technique also is sensitive to flow: When flow moves nuclei rapidly through the planar volumes being excited, the moving nuclei will not be excited as much as the stationary ones. The result is that rapidly moving nuclei exhibit a low intensity in the image. We have seen low intensities from vessels in a live animal increase in intensity when the animal dies (Fig. 3). If this intensity variation with flow could be quantified, one could measure blood flow in the vessel and determine the presence of a plaque from it.

The ability of NMR to directly image a plaque in a given vessel depends on the degree of resolution and the plaque's inherent *in vivo* NMR intensity. Using a whole-body imager, it is optimistic to expect a resolution of 2 mm, which is achieved in the animal imager in a reasonable time. Since the blood flowing next to or around the plaque will have reduced intensity, the contrast between plaque and blood is critically dependent on the NMR intensity of the plaque. If the plaque's intensity is similar to that of the fat in Figure 1, the plaque will appear bright compared with the blood. If the plaque has an inherent low intensity or a long T_1 (with a resulting low intensity), it may be hard to distinguish from the flowing blood. In this case, one might use gating on the EKG to "stop" the flow; the plaque would then appear as a low-intensity spot compared with the blood. Since NMR imaging is electronic, gating would be simple, but obtaining the EKG or its acoustic equivalent during

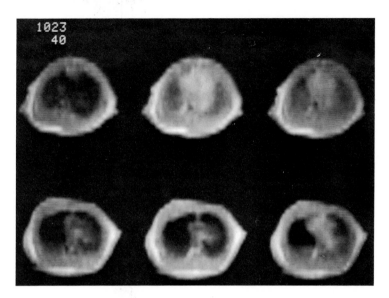

FIG. 3. Three sections through two rats. The first of each row was made when the animals were alive. Note that heart and vessel on the **lower left** are dim. The **upper middle** image was made immediately after death; heart and vessel are brighter due to stopping of motion and blood flow. The **upper right** image was made 1 hr later and demonstrates that intensity is only slightly affected by tissue deterioration. The animal died during the scan of the **lower middle** image. The upper half is live and the lower half dead. The **right** image immediately followed the **middle** image.

imaging may be difficult due to the imposed magnetic fields. The time required to excite a line and receive its associated signal is about 50 msec, about equal to the human heart's low-velocity quiet period.

NMR is appealing because it does not expose the patient to ionizing radiation, but merely to a strong magnetic field, a pulsed radio frequency field, and (in our system) a rapidly changing magnetic field gradient. Published data on the effects of magnetic fields are very diverse (3,4), but a short exposure to the 0.35 T field will not violate the safety standards suggested by the Bureau of Biological Health. The anticipated radio frequency flux through the patient is very close to the OSHA standard of 4 mW/cm^2. A hazard of the rapidly changing field gradients is that the changing magnetic flux might induce currents in the patient; however, one published estimate of the maximum dB/dt that "should not cause biological effects" (3) is twice as high as the level we expect to use. Additional studies are exploring this safety issue.

In conclusion, we think NMR can reliably detect atherosclerosis in two ways; spatially resolved measurement of blood flow and actual imaging of plaques in large vessels. Flow measurement techniques are currently being developed (5). The success of direct imaging will depend on the NMR intensity level of the plaque, the spatial resolution of the image, and the ability to make gated studies. At the exposure levels we will use, moreover, it appears that NMR imaging is not hazardous.

ACKNOWLEDGMENT

This work was funded by Pfizer Inc.

REFERENCES

1. Crooks, L., Hoenninger, J., Arakawa, M., Kaufman, L. McRee, R., and Watts, J. (1979): Tomography of hydrogen with NMR, and the potential for imaging other body constituents. *Proceedings 23rd Annual SPIE*, San Diego.
2. Grover, T., and Singer, J. R. (1971): NMR spin-echo flow measurements. *J. Appl. Physics*, 42:938.
3. Budinger, T. (1979): Thresholds for physiological effects due to RF and magnetic fields used in NMR imaging. *IEEE Trans. Nuclear Science*, NS-26:2821.
4. Tenforde, T. (1978): Proceedings of the Biomagnetic Effects Workshop. LBL-7452.
5. Singer, J. R. (1978): NMR diffusion and flow measurements and an introduction to spin phase graphing. *J. Phys. [E]*, 11:281.

Noninvasive Techniques for Assessment of Atherosclerosis in Peripheral, Carotid, and Coronary Arteries, edited by Thomas F. Budinger, et al. Raven Press, New York 1982.

Commentary

David I. Hoult

Biomedical Engineering and Instrumentation Branch, Division of Research Services, National Institutes of Health, Bethesda, Maryland 20205

An important point brought out by Dr. Waldo Hinshaw, which must be emphasized again and again to the uninitiated, is the immense technical difficulty of nuclear magnetic resonance imaging.

I would like to make a point about the way in which data are presented. There is a great danger for people like myself, who have little clinical experience, to conclude that an image is useful simply because it has a biological significance of some sort. Also, it is too easy to develop a technique of producing artifacts by simply adjusting the contrast and the brightness on the display screen and then carefully removing those artifacts because they are below some arbitrary threshold of significance.

One of Dr. Hinshaw's slides made a nice point. It was produced by a projection reconstruction method, as in CAT scanning, with field gradients applied at different angles at different times—hence, the white artifact in the center. The contrast scale in this picture is black for no signal and white for a large signal, i.e., for the greatest number of hydrogen atoms. (Hydrogen atoms are being observed.) Now, the ventricles appear black, which would perhaps lead a radiologist to suppose that this person were dead. In fact, he is very much alive and well. In this particular image, the pulse repetition interval used in generating the signals was only 0.3 sec, I think, whereas the relaxation rate of pure water is about 2.8 sec. The result was that we did not obtain signals from the C.S.F. in the ventricles, which is essentially pure water. We were not giving it a chance to relax.

On the other hand, for the repetition interval of 0.3 sec, we might presume that there was something seriously wrong with the cerebrospinal fluid in a living patient who showed such a signal. You can see that we have the beginnings of a diagnostic technique that will produce not only images of psychological information. That information, at resolutions of a millimeter in a slice thickness of about 5 mm, I believe, will one day be obtainable from the human head within about 10 to 20 sec.

Regrettably, that scale applies only to protons, hydrogen atoms. Any other nucleus will show a much coarser resolution. You might be able to pick up the

149

phosphorus in quadrants of the heart, for example, but I think we are not going to get better resolution than that within acceptable times.

There are questions of safety. I must put in a plea for an accurate description of the technique. If the system is correctly designed, radiofrequency radiation is not a consideration. There is normally a negligible electric field associated with the alternating magnetic fields that we use. This is not radiation. We operate in a near-field region, hence it is very difficult to describe power in terms of mw/sq cm when no vector is associated with the system.

It is very easy, by misdesigning the system, to produce an electric field that can be lethal. But with a correctly designed system, we have to cope with only an alternating magnetic field. (Incidentally, it is now perfectly possible to get pictures without any field gradient switching.) We must therefore consider the heating effects of the alternating magnetic field when debating safety.

Noninvasive Techniques for Assessment of Atherosclerosis in Peripheral, Carotid, and Coronary Arteries, edited by Thomas F. Budinger, et al. Raven Press, New York 1982.

Nuclear Magnetic Resonance in the Study of Atherosclerosis

Thomas F. Budinger

Donner Laboratory, University of California, Berkeley, California 94720

Techniques for noninvasive evaluation of atherosclerosis in general fall into two categories: (a) the degree of patency or abnormality in flow as measured by X-ray angiography with injected contrast material and ultrasound, and (b) the functional and metabolic consequences of arterial flow on the end organ as measured by ultrasound and radionuclide imaging techniques.

Nuclear magnetic resonance imaging (NMR) has promise as a tool for evaluation of flow, end organ effects of compromised flow, and perhaps of greatest importance, for the evaluation of the composition of the atheromatous plaque. The purpose of this chapter is to present perspectives on the role of NMR in the study of atherosclerosis in these categories:

1. Evaluation of the composition of the arterial wall.
2. Evaluation of flow in arteries.
3. Detection of myocardial ischemia.
4. Measurement of myocardial perfusion.
5. Measurement of tissue oxygen concentration.

ATHEROMATA COMPOSITION

Protons associated with fats have a lower T_1 relaxation time than protons associated with water and tissue fluids. This fact and the extremely short relaxation times of solids such as calcium relative to the T_1 of water or fat lead us to propose NMR as a method for detection of at least fat and calcium (loss of signal) in peripheral arterial tissue (Fig. 1).

Because the heart is in rapid motion and the coronary arteries are surrounded by fat, the potential of the NMR imaging method for evaluating lesions of the major coronary arteries is not great. Nevertheless, NMR studies restricted to the carotid arteries, aorta, and leg arteries are likely to provide a new tool for the study of the influence of diet, exercise, and natural hyperlipemia on the rate of lesion development. They might lead to a method for development of more effective methods

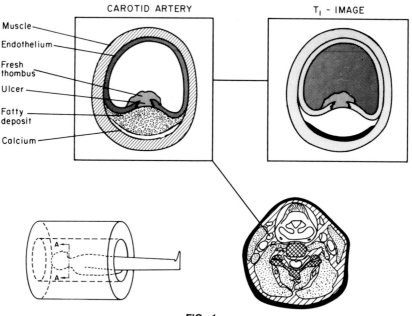

FIG. 1.

of evaluating therapies for advanced atherosclerosis. Preliminary experiments are reported by Crooks et al., *this volume.*

The lack of hazards (1) from fields and imaging strategies used in present instrument designs allow the application of this technique to children and to repeat the evaluation in the same individual as often as required without cumulating harmful health effects. Thus, for the first time the natural history of atherosclerosis can be studied and related to genetic and other factors on an individual basis.

The key limitations are resolution and motion. Though not yet achieved, submillimeter resolution over small regions within the body rather than uniformly high resolution over the entire body appears to be worth pursuing. Should the resolution problems be insurmountable over the next few years, then a slightly invasive method of internal topical magnetic resonance can be applied, at least in animal studies. The essential ideas of this method are shown in Figure 2. The magnetic field of the appropriate value is applied to a region of the body such as a segment of the aorta, and the T_1 relaxation parameter is measured using an rf probe of about 3 mm diameter mounted on a catheter. If the technical problems of noninvasive selected region imaging of < 1 mm are overcome, then NMR will provide information on the tissue composition of diseased arteries. This information can be obtained repeatedly without risk to the patient and can be used in three vital areas: (a) early detection of events in the arterial wall that lead to arteriosclerosis, (b) determination of the rate of progression and regression of disease—that is the natural history from childhood to death, and (c) measurement of the effects of various therapeutic interventions on the change in the size and composition of the lesions.

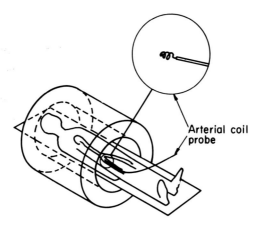

FIG. 2.

FLOW MEASUREMENT

NMR can give relative flow information of blood in vessels from appropriate images wherein the intensity of the signal from moving fluid will vary with the NMR pulse sequence. The capability of NMR to determine flow has been studied (2,3) and recently, the ability of NMR to image, at least qualitatively, the presence and spatial distribution of flow has been shown (4). Nuclei flowing into the imaging volume produce strong signals that compensate for the loss of signals from the nuclei leaving the volume. As a consequence, at low speeds the image intensity reflects a paradoxical enhancement in which laminar flow produces a speed gradient that is seen as a gradual increase in NMR intensities from the center of a vessel toward the walls. This effect, which occurs at speeds of a few centimeters per second, may be important in enhancing the intensity of signals from blood in nearly occluded vessels.

INFARCTION DETECTION

Ischemia is accompanied by an increase in the proton T_1 relaxation time of only about 10% (5,6). Thus, the sensitivity of NMR proton imaging is low for detection of tissue ischemia. The ability of phosphorous NMR spectroscopy to measure the ischemic state of tissue is very high (7). However, because the concentration of phosphorous ATP and creatine phosphate are very low in tissue, the use of P-31 spectroscopy for noninvasive evaluation of the ratio of ATP to creatine phosphate will be limited to large tissue volumes (e.g., 30 cc).

MYOCARDIAL PERFUSION

The proton T_1 relaxation time is lowered in proportion to the amount of para-magnetic ion available for tissue proton interaction (8). The concentration of Mn^{++}, a paramagnetic ion, in the myocardium is proportional to flow a few minutes after injection.

Thus, by imaging the spatial resolution of relaxation time before and after infusion of Mn^{++} it is possible to measure specific volume flow if the input function is also known. The difference in the reciprocals of these relaxation times divided by the normalized time-activity function of Mn^{++} in the left ventricular cavity will give specific volume flow using a model similar to that discussed in Chapter 28 *(this volume)* on emission techniques. This is a suggested method for the NMR measurement of specific volume flow and has not been attempted experimentally.

TISSUE AND BLOOD OXYGEN CONCENTRATION

A major consequence of atherosclerosis is decreased oxygen delivery to tissues. O_2 in the blood can change its T_1 relaxation time. Changes between the right and left ventricular cavities have been noted in ungated NMR human thorax transverse sections.

The influence of hemoglobin on the T_1 was first demonstrated by Singer and Crooks (9) who showed a decrease due to hemoglobin. T_1 was not affected by the oxygen state of the hemoglobin; however, it is decreased by the presence of the paramagnetic O_2. T_2 is also decreased (10). It is still not clear whether T-parameter changes noted *in vivo* or *in vitro* can be related to O_2 content of blood and tissue and how these changes are related to the state of the hemoglobin.

REFERENCES

1. Budinger, T. F. (1981): Nuclear magnetic resonance (NMR) in vivo studies: Known thresholds for health effects. *J. Comput. Assist. Tomogr.*, 5:800–811.
2. Singer, J. R. (1978): NMR diffusion and flow measurements and an introduction to spin phase graphing. *J. Phys. E. Sci. Instrum.*, 11:281–291.
3. Battocletti, J. H., Halbach, R. E., Salles-Cunha, S. X., and Sances, A., Jr. (1981): The NMR blood flowmeter—theory and history. *Med. Phys.*, 8:435–443.
4. Davis, P. L., Kaufman, L., Crooks, L. E., and Margulis, A. R. (1981): NMR characteristics of normal and abnormal rat tissues. In: *Nuclear Magnetic Resonance Imaging in Medicine*, edited by L. Kaufman, L. E. Crooks, and A. R. Margulis, pp. 71–100. Igaku-Shoin Ltd., New York.
5. Williams, E. S., Kaplan, J. I., Thatcher, F., Zimmerman, G., and Knoebel, S. B. (1980): Prolongation of proton spin lattice relaxation times in regionally ischemic tissue from dog hearts. *J. Nucl. Med.*, 21:449–453.
6. Frank, J. A., Feiler, M. A., House, W. V., Lauterbur, P. C., and Jacobson, M. J. (1976): Measurement of proton nuclear magnetic longitudinal relaxation times and water content in infarcted canine myocardium and induced pulmonary injury. *Clin. Res.*, 24:217A. (Abstract).
7. Nunnally, R. L., and Bottomley, P. A. (1981): Assessment of pharmacological treatment of myocardial infarction by phosphorous-31 NMR with surface coils. *Science*, 211:177.
8. Lauterbur, P. C., Mendonca-Diaz, M. H., and Rudin, A. M. (1978): Augmentation of tissue water proton spin-lattice relaxation ratio by in vivo addition of paramagnetic ions. In: *Electrons to Tissue, Frontiers of Biological Energetics*, edited by P. L. Dutton, J. S. Leigh, and A. Scarpa, pp. 752–759. Academic Press, New York.
9. Crooks, L., Hoenninger, J., Arakawa, M., et al. (1979): Tomography of hydrogen with NMR and the potential of imaging other body constituents. *SPIE*, 106:120.
10. Thulborn, K. R., Waterton, J. C., and Radda, G. K. (1981): Proton imaging for in vivo blood flow and oxygen consumption measurements. *J. Magn. Reson.*, 45:188.

Noninvasive Techniques for Assessment of Atherosclerosis in Peripheral, Carotid, and Coronary Arteries, edited by Thomas F. Budinger, et al. Raven Press, New York 1982.

Emission Tomography: An Overview of Instrument Limitations and Potentials

Thomas F. Budinger

Department of Research, Donner Laboratory, University of California, Berkeley, California 94720

DEFINITION AND SCOPE

Emission imaging includes those techniques that involve the observation of γ and X-ray photons emitted from radionuclides (isotopes) injected into the body. The radionuclides are injected frequently as inorganic ions, such as thallium-201 or iodine-123; as gas molecules, such as oxygen-15 or xenon-133; or as labels on organic compounds, such as carbon-11 on palmitic acid, nitrogen-13 on valine, or fluorine-18 on deoxyglucose. Conventional imaging usually involves a projection of the three-dimensional information onto a two-dimensional plane.

Tomography is the act of imaging a slice or section of the object. The slice can be transverse, longitudinal (coronal or sagittal), or oblique. The methods of implementing emission tomography include the invasive technique of thin or thick section radioautography, which involves tissue removal and can be called *in vitro* tomography. The basic difference between radioautography and single photon (γ) or positron (annihilation photon) nuclear medicine techniques is the fact that the latter are noninvasive, except that a radioactive tracer is injected or inhaled.

This chapter presents an overview of the instrumentation and strategies presently employed to implement emission tomography, catalogues the major areas where problems or limitations exist, and, finally, discusses some potential outcomes that might be realized with state-of-the-art and improved instrumentation. The important conclusions are that needs exist for improvement in detector sensitivity, in ability to image larger regions than provided by single sections for the thorax, in data compression, and in display of easily interpretable results.

In addition to the emission instrumentation improvements, isotope production devices, ranging from cyclotrons to generators, are in need of refinements and innovations for automation of radiopharmaceutical preparation. Another area of needed device and methodology improvements for development of emission tomography involves strategies for evaluating the physiological mechanisms of radiopharmaceutical distribution. The emphasis here is on tomography; however, in situations where the target-to-nontarget activity is high (i.e., 10:1), important non-invasive imaging studies and developments can be made with projection imaging.

SINGLE PHOTON TOMOGRAPHY

The types of devices and general idea of single photon tomography are shown in Fig. 1. The earliest device, that of Kuhl and Edwards (1), employed a rectilinear scanner comprised of a collimator and NaI(T1) crystal scintillator with a phototube detector. Photon count information from multiple linear positions and angles was gathered in a way somewhat similar to the early X-ray-computed tomograph invented a decade later, except that using the former, single events, rather than photon fluence, were detected.

Initially, the reconstruction algorithm was simple superposition with an evolution to versions of iterative arithmetic optimization techniques. Early devices provided only single sections. Area detectors, such as the Anger camera, were used for tomography beginning about 1973 by rotating phantoms or patients in front of the camera (2–5). From this approach evolved prototype instruments that rotate around the patient (6,7). The limitations in the use of single photons for tomography are the poor efficiency (system sensitivity) of the detection schemes and the mathematical difficulties in reconstruction of data emitted from portions of the body with variable attenuation coefficients. The seriousness of the problem of sensitivity is exemplified by the fact that only a few events/sec/μCi are detected by the Anger-type area detector; 20 plus min of data collection are thus needed to give transverse thoracic sections which warrant some confidence in the statistical validity of the

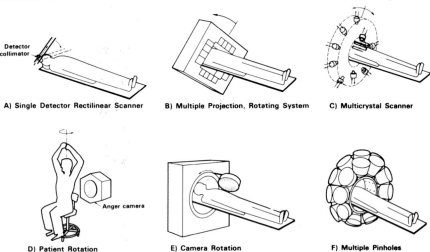

A) Single Detector Rectilinear Scanner   B) Multiple Projection, Rotating System   C) Multicrystal Scanner

D) Patient Rotation   E) Camera Rotation   F) Multiple Pinholes

FIG. 1. Six techniques for emission computed tomography using single photon (γ) radionuclides. **Upper row**: single section devices. **Lower row**: area devices. The multiple pinhole scheme (F) has not been implemented, but conveys the need for multiple angles and a large detector area to improve sensitivity.

image data. These problems were analyzed in the context of thallium-201-gated computed tomography in 1977 (8) and other radionuclides in 1979 (9). The ratio between the number of resolution elements and the data required for achieving quantitatively reliable results can be calculated as shown in Figs. 2 through 4.

A similar problem of low sensitivity exists for the Anger tomoscanner (11). This problem motivated exploration of coded apertures commencing with the Fresnel zone plate in 1972 (12) and digital tomography methods in 1975 (13). Heart studies were done on animals in 1976 (14). In 1974, the first coded aperture studies emphasizing multiple pinholes were applied to humans (15) and discarded due to the nonquantitative nature of data from limited angular views. More recently, Kirch and Vogel (16) have shown some efficacy for the diagnostic use of a seven-pinhole system, which is the subject for current multi-institutional clinical trials.

A coded aperture approach to myocardial imaging involves a multitude of pinholes arranged in a fashion so as to optimize the data reconstruction. The main limitation of coded aperture techniques, whether they are digitized Anger tomoscanner methods or time varying aperture arrays (17), is the problem of limited angular views. This is similar to trying to solve a mathematical problem with fewer equations than unknowns. Coded aperture schemes that surround the patient are required to overcome the limited angle problem.

Accurate single-photon tomography requires a device placing enough detector surface around the body to make imaging of isotope behavior in the myocardium

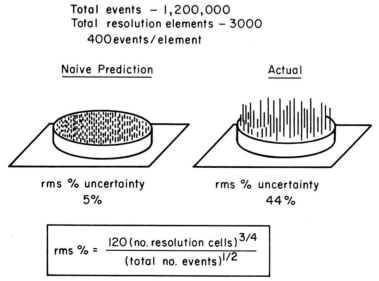

Total events − 1,200,000
Total resolution elements − 3000
400 events/element

Naive Prediction   Actual

rms % uncertainty   rms % uncertainty
5%   44%

$$rms\ \% = \frac{120\,(\text{no. resolution cells})^{3/4}}{(\text{total no. events})^{1/2}}$$

FIG. 2. Relationship between expected uncertainty for data collected from a two-dimensional image and actual uncertainty when a two-dimensional section is reconstructed from multiple projections.

$$\frac{\sigma\,C}{C} = \sqrt{\frac{1.4\,(\text{total cells})^{3/2}}{\text{total counts}}}$$

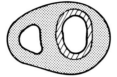

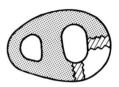

Subendocardial ischemia of 30%	Anterolateral infarction with marginal ischemia of 70%
Events per slice: 300,000	55,000
Total for 4 slices: 1,200,000	220,000
Total for 7 cardiac phases: 8,400,000	1,540,000

FIG. 3. Statistics needed for reconstruction. Prediction of the number of events needed to achieve quantitative image information under conditions of subendocardial ischemia and transmural infarction (8).

practical in a few minutes or even a few seconds. Three approaches to this solution are:

1. Kuhl's Mark IV device (18), which has a sensitivity close to the positron devices for head scanning but needs modification for thorax scanning and is limited to single sections.

2. Union Carbide's system for single sections (Fig. 1C), which achieves a sensitivity that is competitive with the positron systems; however, this device undersamples in angle and gives aliasing artifacts.

3. These problems could be avoided by the theoretical device shown in Fig. 1F, which was suggested by the author a few years ago as a brute force approach to overcoming the sensitivity problem as well as the need for multiple sections.

Single photon tomography engineering is likely to continue to gather momentum, and interpretable brain and lower extremity blood flow observations can be made presently from single section devices; however, without clever schemes whereby multiple sections with high sensitivities can be obtained, it is unlikely that important medical and scientific advances in myocardial disease will benefit from this instrumentation development.

Another problem of tomographic imaging of the thorax involves the reconstruction strategy. The linear attenuation coefficient varies in the thorax between 0.05 and

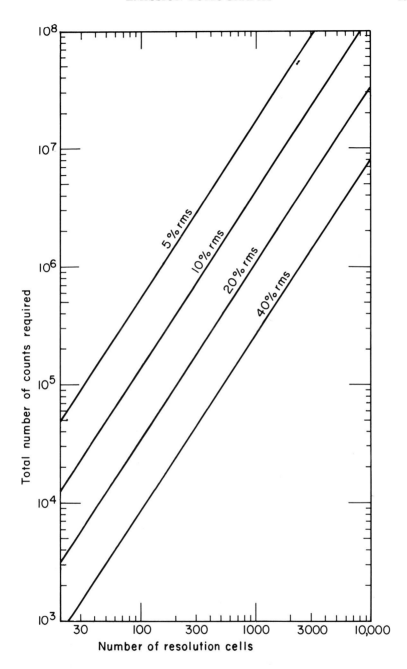

FIG. 4. Relationship among the number of counts needed in order to achieve a specific rms uncertainty for images with various resolutions (10).

0.3 for ^{99m}Tc. In emission tomography, we seek the position and strength of isotope distributions, and we must include in our strategy some method to account for the variable attenuation between those unknown sources and the detectors at various angles. This task is far more difficult than that of X-ray tomography, wherein the source position and strength are known at all times and only the attenuation coefficient needs to be determined.

The methods for attenuation compensating have been the subject of intense investigations by a few groups, and the results are summarized in two extensive discussions (19,20). The importance of such methods is illustrated in Fig. 5. Projections from a uniform disc of activity were used to reconstruct that activity without compensation for attenuation. There are a number of good methods for attenuation compensation in single photon emission tomography under conditions of constant attenuation (19–21), and a simple general technique exists for compensation in positron tomography (18,22). The only acceptable method known for variable attenuation coefficient is the weighted least squares method (2,20). Implementation of this technique in clinical work will require dedication of medium to large computers (e.g., VAX 11/780, CDC 7600) with special purpose hardware processors. Data multiplexing is the bottleneck for hardware implementation at present.

POSITRON TOMOGRAPHY

A positron-emitting radionuclide, such as ^{11}C, ^{13}N, ^{15}O, ^{38}K, ^{52}Fe, ^{52m}Mn, or ^{82}Rb, is an atom whose nucleus has a deficiency of neutrons. The forces of nature prompt this nucleus to change one of its protons to a neutron, which is accomplished

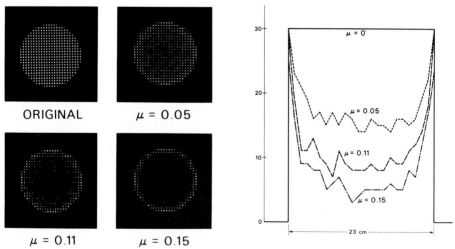

FIG. 5. Impact of reconstructing emission data without taking into account compensation for attenuation in single photon-computed tomography. Attenuation coefficient of 0.11 corresponds approximately to that for 511 keV photons; μ = 0.15 is the attenuation coefficient experienced by low energy isotopes, such as technetium-99m and I-123. Profiles of activity distribution in the reconstructed disks are shown on the **right**.

by the release of a positron (electron with a plus charge) and a neutrino. The positron travels a few millimeters in tissue and, as it slows, interacts with an electron. The matter and antimatter interaction results in annihilation of the masses of the positron and electron with a resultant release of energy in the form of two photons with energies of 511 keV and directions of travel 180° opposite each other.

These annihilation photons are detected by scintillation crystals just as if they were single photons; however, a true event is recorded when the two annihilation photons are simultaneously detected by opposing detectors (Fig. 6). Because of the presence of out-of-plane activity, scatter in tissue, and detector inefficiencies, only 0.5 to 1% of the detected photons contribute to the true coincident events. Accidental coincidences occur when photons from different positron-electron annihilations are

FATES OF ANNIHILATION PHOTONS

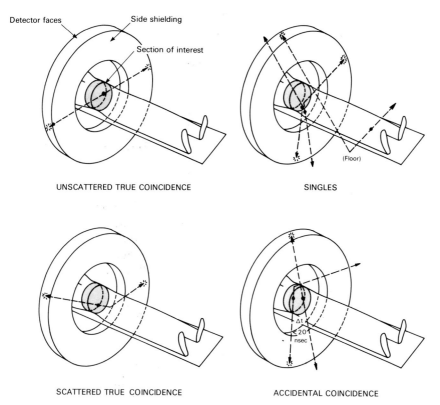

FIG. 6. Only a few of the annihilation photons from positron-emitting isotopes escape the body unscattered in directions that can be detected by the positron emission tomograph. Advances in instrumentation involve improving the solid angle for detection of true unscattered coincident events and avoiding detection of scattered coincidences or accidental coincidences, each of which comprises 10 to 20% of the events detected under high-count-rate imaging situations.

detected by chance within the time coincidence window. Scattered coincidences occur when both detected photons originate from the same positron, but one or both have scattered in tissue. Typically, 10 to 20% of detected coincident events are accidental events, and 10 to 20% are scattered events. To obtain quantitative information, the imaging procedure must correct for these sources of error.

The instrument concepts for positron tomography are shown in Fig. 7. The concept of transverse section tomography was first embodied in a positron device comprising 32 sodium iodide crystals and phototubes surrounding a patient's head [built at Brookhaven National Laboratory in 1962 by Rankowitz et al. (23)]. The first practical positron emission transaxial tomograph (PETT) systems were described by Ter-Pogossian et al. (24,25). Cho (26) presented a ring design comprised of 64 crystals in 1976.

Another positron ring device, built in Sweden, has 95 crystals and is designed to wobble in order to achieve improved sampling (27). Also noteworthy are the improvements by Thompson of the original 32-crystal Brookhaven system, which is being used for brain blood flow imaging by Yamamoto and coworkers (28). A 64-crystal bismuth germanate ring system has recently been completed by that group. The largest ring is the Donner 280-crystal system designed specifically for myocardial imaging (29).

Devices for multiple transverse sections using positron emitters include both the positron camera and multicrystal rings (Fig. 7C–F). The Massachusetts General Hospital positron camera of Brownell and Burnham has been modified to perform a 180° rotation for transverse section computed tomography (22). Two large field-of-view Anger cameras were modified by Muehllehner and co-workers (30) to rotate around the patient, and the wire chamber device of Perez-Mendez was redesigned for positron tomography (31).

Multilayer ring devices designed by the Washington University group include PETT IV (32) and, more recently, PETT V, which is a circular configuration of crystals wherein the axial position of an event is determined from the relative proportion of light arriving at photo detectors at each end of the crystal (33). Other multilayer ring systems include a new version of the ORTEC ECAT comprised of two octagonal rings; a wraparound version of the Brownell-Burnham camera, designed by L. Carroll of Cyclotron Corporation; a system using multiple layers of cesium fluoride crystals at Washington University (PETT VI), discussed by M. Ter-Pogossian (*this volume*); and a very large system comprised of three layers of bismuth germanate (BGO) crystals, designed by the Donner Laboratory group.

The evolution of these systems has been toward increasing sensitivity, decreasing the fraction of accidental coincidences and scattered coincidences, and achieving a geometry that will allow information from the full three-dimensional volume to be collected after a single injection.

Sensitivity

The sensitivity of a ring system is dependent on the area and efficiency of detector crystals and the ring radius. Crystal efficiency is dependent on the density and

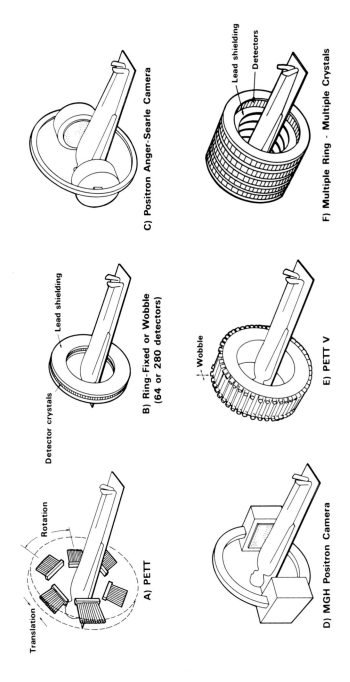

FIG. 7. Six positron emission instrumentation concepts.

atomic number. The applicable equation and a sample calculation for BGO are given below. Bismuth germanate has a 2-to-3 time advantage over NaI(T1) in efficiency for PETT applications (34). A second disadvantage of NaI(T1) is the fact that this hygroscopic material has a finite lifetime due to crystal deterioration. The disadvantages of BGO are lower light yield and higher cost at present relative to NaI(T1). The improved photopeak efficiency and stability of BGO outweigh these disadvantages. Cesium fluoride has far superior timing than NaI(T1) or BGO and thus might become the best detector if the packaging technology can overcome the hygroscopic nature of CsF.

SENSITIVITY

$$N_T = \frac{\rho S N_o \times A \, (e^{-2\mu L})(\epsilon^2)}{2 \times 4\pi R^2}$$

where

N_o = 37,0000 events sec^{-1} Ci^{-1}
ρ = number μCi cm^{-1} of a line source parallel to the ring axis
S = shielding gap
A = detector area = 2 RS
μ = 0.098 cm^{-1}
L = thickness of the attenuating medium
ϵ = single crystal efficiency
Example for human head: e^{-L} = 0.2
R = 30 cm
ρ = 300 μCi
ϵ = 0.8
N_T = 47,360 true coincidences/sec

Resolution

Three factors which degrade resolution are: (a) a slight deviation from 180° of $\pm 0.25°$ for the annihilation photons, (b) the range of positrons in tissue, and (c) geometric detector sampling characteristics. The deviation from 180° leads to an error of 1 to 2 mm full width half max (FWHM) for typical geometries.

The range of positrons in tissue is a very fundamental limit to the spatial resolution of positron imaging systems. Figure 8 shows the point spread function for positron emitters whose energies are 3.3 MeV (^{82}Rb), 1.9 MeV (^{68}Ga), and 1 MeV (^{11}C) from recent experiments of Derenzo (35). Note that the FWHM is small but that the contribution of the "tails" can be expected to cause image blurring with high resolution systems.

The third factor in emission tomography resolution is geometric sampling. The well-known Nyquist sampling theorem requires data to be sampled with a spacing one-half that of the expected resolution; however, some geometries give a sampling that is not uniform over the image region (36). Thus, the point spread function

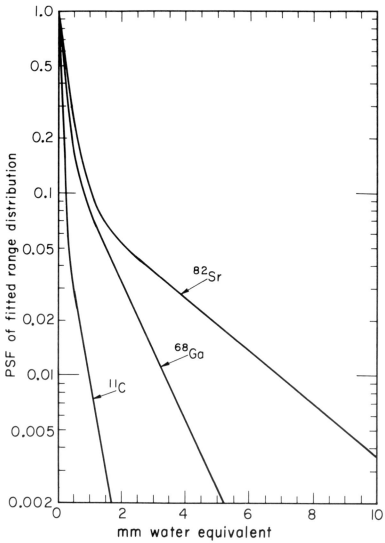

FIG. 8. Fit to data collected by Derenzo (39), showing the point spread due to positron range in water.

varies locally, as well as regionally. To achieve uniform sampling, as well as finer sampling than allowed from crystal spacing, some translational motion has been employed (37) and is used in PETT V (38) and the Swedish system (27). If rapid dynamic studies are done on the heart, radionuclide concentration and the organ position changes are great over a period of less than 1 sec, and wobbling the imaging system has definite disadvantages. On the other hand, the only way to overcome the aliasing problem associated with irregular or coarse sampling is to obtain finer samples, either by using more detectors or a location scheme in large crystals, such as the PETT V design (36). For multilayer systems, sampling along the Z-axis presents another source of variation in the point spread function, as well as in the spatial sensitivity.

There is a close connection between spatial resolution and detection or quantitation of diminished uptake, as shown in Fig. 9. It should be recognized that a system with a spatial resolution of 10 mm FWHM will necessarily have a quantitative resolution cell approximately 20 mm FWHM.

Optimization of Instrumentation for Emission Tomographs

Optimization of emission tomographic instrumentation involves a strategy of maximizing the signal-to-noise and resolution for a given dose to the patient. The important parameters are crystal efficiency, detector time resolution, coupling geometry, shielding thickness and depth, and sampling interval. Shielding configuration plays an important role in minimizing the contributions of scatter and accidental coincidences.

Whereas the problem of optimization of a single-section device seems well in hand (39), a method for a multislice device is still under development (40,41). As emphasized by Brownell et al. (40), we are presently a factor of 100 from the theoretical limit in sensitivity; however, to increase the solid angle in order to improve sensitivity means diminished shielding, and thus scattered and accidental coincidences will increase. Accidental coincidence contribution can be reduced by development of faster detector systems, and scatter can be extracted to some extent by iterative calculations.

RADIONUCLIDE AVAILABILITY

Isotope production via reactors and cyclotrons temporarily diminished as a problem 10 years ago, when most of nuclear medicine centered around the use of Tc-99m pertechnetate. There is currently a resurgence of interest in a broad spectrum of single photon and positron-emitting radionuclides. Not all positron emitters require a cyclotron for their immediate availability, as many can be obtained from generators. For example, ^{68}Ga ($t_{1/2}$ = 68 min) is obtained from a long-lived ^{68}Ge parent, while ^{82}Rb ($t_{1/2}$ = 76 sec) is obtained by passing 2% NaCl through a small column of alumina on which is adsorbed ^{82}Sr ($t_{1/2}$ = 25 days), which is the radioactive parent of ^{82}Rb (Fig. 10) (42). Some other generators of importance to positron tomography include ^{52}Fe-^{52m}Mn and ^{122}Xe-^{122}I.

The task of isotope production, whether single photon or positron emitter, is only one aspect of radiopharmaceutical development. A second aspect is radiopharmaceutical preparation, which can become the most significant roadblock for some potential applications, e.g., ^{11}C-labeling of 1-valine or preparation of Ca-antagonists with positron labels of high specific activity.

Instrumentation is needed to automate syntheses of radiopharmaceuticals, because the half-life is frequently short relative to the usual synthesis times. Some cumulative

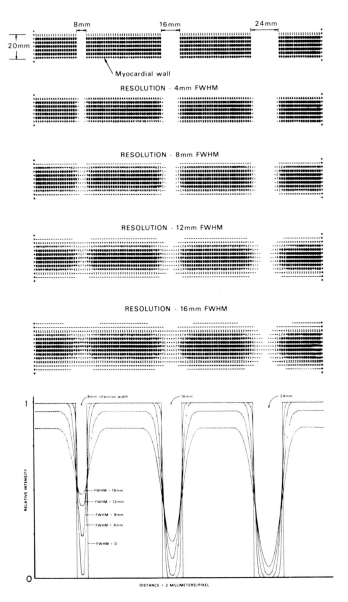

FIG. 9. Images expected for transmural infarctions of various sizes (**top**), imaged by systems with resolution varying from 4 to 16 mm (FWHM). Note that the quantitative resolution size is twice the FWHM resolution, as one would expect from the definition of FWHM.

hand and body radiation burden is being assumed by chemists and technicians, particularly in the more complicated syntheses. An example where rapid synthesis methods can lead to more handling is in the Strecker reaction for preparation of amino acids labeled with ^{11}C. A modification of this reaction was needed to ac-

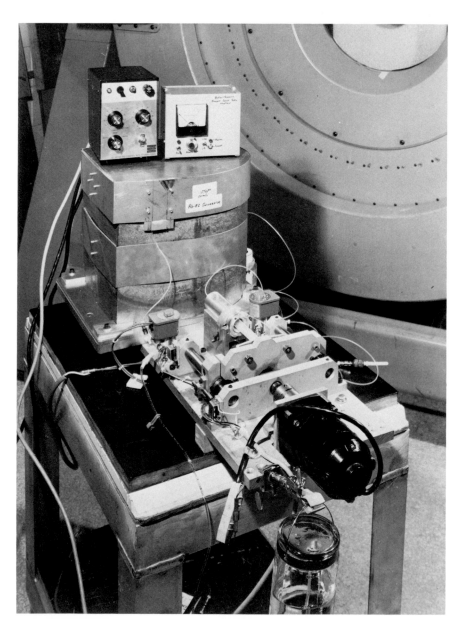

FIG. 10. The Donner strontium-rubidium generator, which can deliver over 100 mCi as a bolus injection at 5-min intervals, consists of a small ion exchange column on which is adsorbed strontium-82. Rubidium-82 is eluted by 2% NaCl (42).

complish the final hydrolysis in a few min, rather than the usual 12-hr acid hydrolysis. To accomplish this, the amino nitrile is placed in a bomb for high pressure and elevated temperature hydrolysis. To avoid radiation exposure the amino acid synthesis requires automation. Analogous situations exist for practically every radiopharmaceutical obtained from cyclotrons and generators. Even single photon labeling requires some innovations to minimize radiation exposure to personnel.

The third aspect involves understanding what happens to the label after injection into the patient and what physiological conditions alter the distribution. For example, after injection of ^{13}N-ammonia, what are the rates of incorporation of ^{13}N into glutamine, and how does the distribution change if the intracellular pH changes? Under what conditions can we expect ^{18}F-deoxyglucose to accumulate in the heart, and how do we separate metabolic extraction from flow? These are examples of areas of research and careful characterization of radiopharmaceutical distribution that must accompany instrument development.

POTENTIAL OF EMISSION TOMOGRAPHY FOR ASSESSMENT OF ATHEROSCLEROSIS

Physiological Principles

Having discussed some of the basic instrumentation and chemical concepts, we turn to the major physiological objectives of this volume. As can be seen from Fig. 4, the number of events required for accurate imaging of 1- to 2-mm lesions is enormous. Further, it is not reasonable to expect a spatial resolution better than 2 mm FWHM from considerations of the range of positrons and the $\pm 0.25°$ deviation from 180° in line of flight of annihilation pairs. Thus, in the applications below, we note techniques whereby the absence or presence of atherosclerosis is inferred mainly from flow through large arteries of interest or from measurement of perfusion through the target organ, i.e., brain, myocardium, leg muscles, etc.

The basic principle that underlies most of the techniques for ascertaining flow and metabolism in emission tomography is the law of conservation of material. In words, the change in amount of a substance with time q(t) is equal to the input rate minus the amount leaving the tissue by flow and through radioactive decay:

$$\frac{dq(t)}{dt} = FA(t) - \frac{F}{V} q(t) - \lambda q(t) \qquad (i)$$

Here q is the amount in the tissue, F is flow, F/V is specific volume flow, A is the arterial input concentration, and λ is the decay constant. It is interesting to note that this equation is precisely the Fick principle and the starting point for derivations of the Stewart-Hamilton or Kety-Schmidt equations if radioactive decay q(t) is neglected and we relate amount/volume [q(t)/V], to output concentration [B(t)], as in the equation

$$\frac{dq(t)}{dt} = F[A(t) - B(t)] \tag{ii}$$

The Kety-Schmidt equation is used extensively in nuclear cardiology for myocardial, skeletal muscle, and skin blood flow using coronary or tissue injection of xenon or krypton as diffusible but inert tracers.

This basic conservation equation is now being applied in nuclear medicine with new instrumentation for noninvasive three-dimensional measurement of brain flow, myocardial flow, and flow to the extremities. In addition, these principles underlie the methods for quantitating amino acid metabolism, oxygen utilization, fatty acid metabolism, and glucose utilization. These latter capabilities for noninvasive studies comprise the unique advantages of positron tomography.

For a substance that accumulates in tissue and does not diffuse freely through tissue, flow is estimated from the relation: Amount present in an organ = flow × extraction × sum of input concentration, or:

$$q(T) = F \cdot E \int_o^T A(t)dt \tag{iii}$$

This relation assumes that the amount that accumulates in tissue on the first pass is proportional to flow, and that the integral of the input concentration can be accurately determined. One of the exciting aspects of positron tomography is the fact that this input function can be ascertained with new instrumentation that has sufficient sensitivity and sampling speed to allow the dynamic input function to be ascertained by observing data over the region of interest in the left ventricle (Fig. 11) or over the carotid or femoral arteries.

Thus, flow × extraction is obtained from Eq. iii:

$$F \cdot E = \frac{q(T)}{\int_o^T A(t)dt}$$

There are five types of input functions that can be programmed to match the imaging objectives with the radionuclides and instrumentation available: (a) bolus infusion; (b) variable infusion (43); (c) programmed exponentially decreasing infusion (44); (d) programmed exponentially increasing infusion; and (e) constant infusion.

Methods of controlling the denominator in Eq. iii are presently being explored by a number of groups (43,44). As an example, we show how the measurements of specific volume flow in brain, heart, or peripheral tissues can be made using the basic conservation-of-material equation. Note that at equilibrium, achieved through programmed infusion that can be exponentially decreasing or constant, a steady state is reached at which the differential change $[dq(t)/dt]$ equals 0. Thus, in Eq. i, we have:

$$0 = FA(t) - \frac{F}{V} q(t) - \lambda q(t)$$

and

$$q(t) = \frac{FA(t)}{\frac{F}{V} + \lambda} \qquad (iv)$$

This method of evaluating flow from equilibrium imaging has been applied to brain blood flow evaluation using krypton (45) and ^{15}O using the MGH positron camera (46).

If we note that the quantity in the tissue is equal to the concentration times the volume, $q = CV$, where C is the tissue concentration:

$$F = \lambda \frac{C}{A} \cdot V + \frac{F}{V} \cdot \frac{C}{A} V \qquad (v)$$

which reduces to

$$\frac{F}{V} = \frac{\lambda}{(\frac{A}{C} + 1)}$$

Thus specific volume flow can be determined from the ratio of arterial to tissue concentration, which is determined as illustrated in Fig. 11.

Once flow is known, then use of Eq. iii with a metabolically active substance can give a measure of extraction.

By observing concentration changes as a function of time, it is possible to infer metabolism, as is done with ^{11}C-palmitic acid disappearance from the heart, or O_2 utilization using $^{15}O_2$.

CAROTID ARTERIES

Three techniques of emission tomography applied to carotid arteries are presented. Direct imaging of injured and atheromatous carotid arteries has been done using labeled platelets. In single photon studies, indium has been used (47), and in positron emission tomography, ^{68}Ga has been used (48).

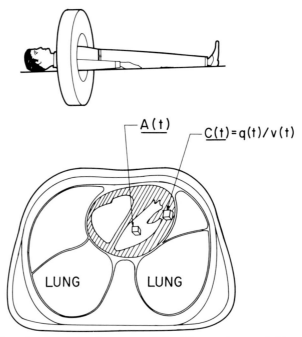

FIG. 11. Arterial input function, as well as myocardial uptake, can be sampled by a region of interest in the gated transverse section.

Static or dynamic imaging of carotid arteries using an intravascular label, such as ^{11}CO-hemoglobin or ^{82}Rb, is possible but is less sensitive than other methods of evaluating flow through the carotid arteries.

A third method that has high potential as a sensitive indicator of the consequences of a particular carotid lesion involves measurement of brain blood flow noninvasively. Though the blood flow being measured will be a reflection of both carotid and cerebral artery disease, end organ blood flow assessment using diffusible tracers is a sensitive technique for evaluating the biological consequences of obstructive vessel disease. Methods of evaluating brain blood flow with emission tomography involve use of diffusible radioisotope tracers: the gases Xe or Kr or labeled iodoantipyrine for single photon tomography; and ^{15}O-labeled water, ^{11}C-labeled alcohols, ^{11}C-acetylene, or ^{13}N-nitrous oxide for positron tomography.

CORONARY ARTERIES AND MYOCARDIUM

As reviewed above, the anatomical distribution of coronary arteries and presence of atheromata are inferred from measurement of tissue perfusion or metabolism. Noninvasive imaging methods of evaluating myocardial perfusion have been the objective of much activity in positron tomography (43,49–53). Recent work was discussed by Drs. Ter-Pogossian and Strauss for the fields of positron tomography and single photon tomography.

Our work at Donner Laboratory has been directed toward validation of ^{82}Rb as a flow indicator. The rationale for this emphasis is that ^{82}Rb is readily available and can be used to normalize other studies for flow, such as fatty acid and amino acid metabolism. The instrument we developed for the thorax has 280 crystals (Fig. 12), and since each crystal is in coincidence with 105 opposing crystals, we can image 14,700 (280/2 × 105) coincidence lines almost simultaneously. The resolution is 9 mm for the images of Fig. 13, which is a transverse section showing the uptake of ^{82}Rb in the normal myocardium at rest and exercise. Implementation of the principles of equilibrium imaging (discussed above) with positron tomography is shown in a patient study (Fig. 14). The constant infusion method of Eq. iv and the bolus techniques of Eq. iii are now being validated using microspheres in acute studies in dogs. Our most recent work demonstrates the need for gating if one wishes to obtain arterial blood concentration [A(t)] without contamination of the volume of interest from myocardial activity entering that region during part of the cardiac cycle (Fig. 15).

These examples illustrate the potential role of positron tomography in early detection of coronary artery disease using exercise versus nonexercise imaging and the role of positron tomography in measuring specific volume flow. The objective of myocardial infarction sizing seems to be well in hand if positron tomography is used. Infarctions of 2 cc can be reliably detected, and lesions as small as 0.7 cc have been detected in dogs. However, the practical aspects of implementing a high-speed, gated instrument in the coronary care unit require more innovative engineering-physics developments.

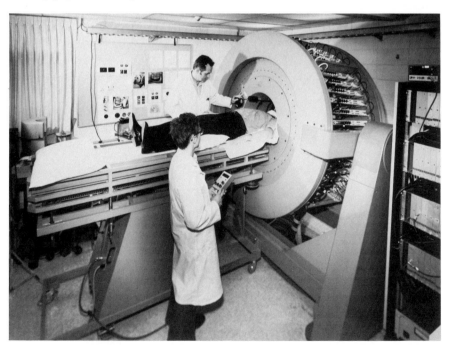

FIG. 12. The Donner 280-crystal positron tomograph.

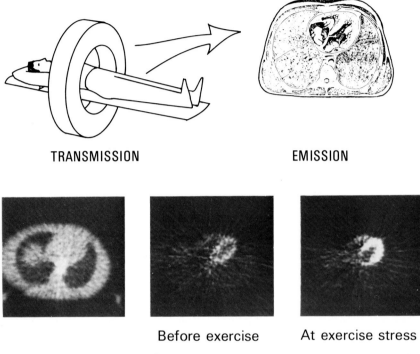

TRANSMISSION   EMISSION

Before exercise   At exercise stress

FIG. 13. Approximately 600,000 events were collected in 5 min after injection of 20 mCi of Rb-82 before exercise. Twenty min after supine exercise, 1 million events were collected under the same injection conditions. Ratio of uptake: 1.7.

PERIPHERAL ARTERIES

One of the strong candidates for noninvasive evaluation of peripheral artery disease is positron tomography used with the equilibrium imaging technique for measurement of blood flow in the limbs. Preliminary studies by Brownell and associates (55) have yielded evidence that images obtained during continuous inhalation of $CO^{15}O_2$ (which converts to $H_2^{15}O$ in the lungs) will give a sensitive measure of the perfusion to the lower limbs.

CONCLUSIONS

The major and nearly unique advantage of emission tomography over other modalities is that it provides a noninvasive method of measuring the spatial distribution of tissue perfusion and metabolism.

During the course of this account on instrumentation and physiological topics relevant to noninvasive imaging with isotopes, a number of limitations were mentioned, and these and related topics for future development are recounted here:

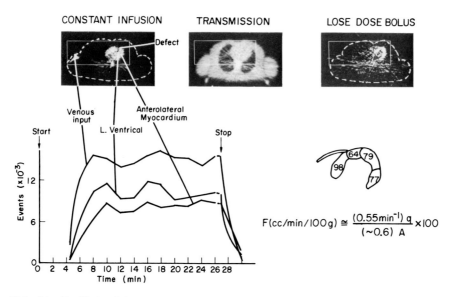

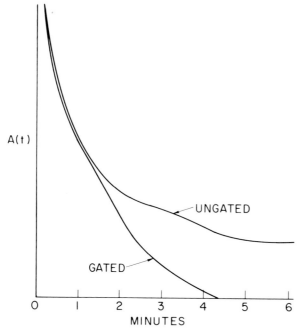

FIG. 14. Equilibrium infusion study with Rb-82 on a patient with an old anteroseptal infarct.

FIG. 15. Illustration of arterial concentration curve for Rb-82, obtained from a region of interest as shown in Fig. 11. Departure of the ungated curve from the gated curve is due to myocardial activity entering the ventricular region of interest during systole.

1. Sensitivity of single photon devices is more than 10 times less than positron instruments. Thus, it is difficult to obtain good resolution data within practical examination time limits.

2. The present sensitivity of positron tomographs also limits realization of the full potential of performing dynamic emission tomography.

3. It is unrealistic to expect resolution better than 2 mm FWHM, due to the high dosage necessary for statistically valid data and other physical considerations.

4. Sampling techniques that require motion of the detectors, while clever and convenient, present problems of inconsistent data when imaging the beating heart and radionuclide activity that rapidly changes in the field of view.

5. Single section tomographic devices for both positron and single photon modes have application in brain, carotid, and femoral artery studies in which some end-organ flow distribution can be sampled by a single slice; however, multisection machines are needed for imaging the heart.

6. Multisection machines for the thorax must be gated to allow the full potential of quantitating the input arterial function in flow and metabolic studies.

7. Data control and display present enormous problems for a multisection gated machine. Consider a study wherein data from nine sections are taken for eight intervals of the cardiac cycle at time intervals of 15 s for 5 min: $9 \times 8 \times 4 \times 5 = 1,440$ reconstructions and displays. Data compression schemes, such as reconstruction of functional images depicting mean transit time (54), might reduce this by a factor of 20, but we are left with the problem of displaying 72 sections in a fashion that can be interpreted. This problem is shared by the Mayo Clinic dynamic spatial reconstructor, discussed by Dr. Erik Ritman (*this volume*).

8. Radiopharmaceutical development can be improved by development of rapid synthesis techniques and automation of radioactive labeling in a manner that will minimize radiation dose to chemists and technicians.

9. The immediate objective of emission tomography is to quantitate the concentration of a radionuclide in a volume of interest without interference of activity from over- and underlying regions. Though it is now possible to extract data from volumes (1 to 4 cc) of interest anywhere in the body, an important problem of local superposition of physiological compartments remains. Each volume of interest represents activity in three compartments: intravascular space, interstitial fluid space, and intracellular space. To sort out the contribution of activity from each compartment, kinetic modeling is used. But most kinetic modeling requires dynamic data. Thus we are led to the conclusion that new developments are needed in rapid dynamic emission tomography.

The summary conclusion of this chapter is that the most important objectives for new developments are improvements in sensitivity, timing, resolution, sampling speed, and data processing for detectors, and in new schemes for rapid and automatic labeling of radiopharmaceuticals and radionuclide delivery from cyclotrons.

ACKNOWLEDGMENTS

The work presented in this chapter evolved from discussions with Drs. S. Derenzo, R. Huesman, L. Sherman, B. Moyer, and Y. Yano from Donner Laboratory, and with Dr. M. Ter-Pogossian of Washington University and Dr. G. Brownell of Harvard University. Support for this work was provided by the National Heart, Lung, and Blood Institute and the United States Department of Energy. Manuscript assistance was given by Ms. Mary Graham and Ms. Linda Lutgens.

REFERENCES

1. Kuhl, D. E., and Edwards, R. O. (1963): Image separation radioisotope scanning. *Radiology*, 80:653.
2. Budinger, T. F., and Gullberg, G. T. (1974): Three-dimensional reconstruction in nuclear medicine by iterative least squares and Fourier transform techniques. *IEEE Trans Nucl Sci*, NS-21(3):2.
3. Oppenheim, B. E. (1974): More accurate algorithms for iterative three-dimension reconstruction. *IEEE Trans Nucl Sci*, NS-21(3):72.
4. Kay, D. B, Keyes, J. W., Jr., and Simon, W. (1974): Radionuclide tomographic image reconstruction using Fourier transform techniques. *J. Nucl. Med.*, 15:981.
5. Budinger, T. F., and Gullberg, G. T. (1977): Transverse section reconstruction of gamma-ray emitting radionuclides in patients. In: *Reconstruction Tomography in Diagnostic Radiology and Nuclear Medicine*, edited by M. M. Ter-Pogossian, M. E. Phelps, G. L. Brownell, and J. R. Cox Jr., pp. 315-342. University Park Press, Baltimore.
6. Keyes, J. W., Orlandea, N., Heetderks, W. J., Leonard, P. F., and Rogers, W. L. (1977): The humongotron—A scintillation camera transaxial tomograph. *J. Nucl. Med.*, 18:381.
7. Jaszczak, R. J., Murphy, P. H., Huard, D., and Burdine, J. A. (1977): Radionuclide emission computed tomography of the head wtih ^{99m}Tc and a scintillation camera. *J. Nucl. Med.*, 18:373.
8. Budinger, T. F., Cahoon, J. L., Derenzo, S. E., Gullberg, G. T., Moyer, B. R., and Yano, Y. (1977): Three-dimensional imaging of the myocardium with radionuclides. *Radiology*, 125:433.
9. Burdine, J. A., Murphy, P. H., and DePuey, E. G. (1979): Radionuclide computed tomography of the body using routine radiopharmaceuticals. II. Clinical applications. *J. Nucl. Med.*, 20:208.
10. Budinger, T. F., Derenzo, S. E., Gullberg, G. T., Greenberg, W. L., and Huesman, R. H. (1977): Emission computer assisted tomography with single-photon and positron annihilation photon emitters. *J. Comput. Assist. Tomogr.*, 1:131.
11. Anger, H. O. (1967): The scintillation camera for radioisotope localization. In: *Radioisotope in der Lokalisations—diagnostik*, edited by G. Hoffman and K. E. Sheer, pp.18–21. FK Schattauer-Verlag, Stuttgart.
12. Barrett, H. H. (1972): Fresnel zone plate imaging in nuclear medicine. *J. Nucl. Med.*, 13:382.
13. Budinger, T. F., and MacDonald, B. (1975): Reconstruction of the Fresnel-coded gamma camera images by digital computer. *J. Nucl. Med.*, 16:309.
14. Holman, B. L., Idoine, J. D., Sos, T. A., Tancrell, R., and DeMeester, G. (1977): Tomographic scintigraphy of regional myocardial perfusion. *J. Nucl. Med.*, 18:764.
15. Mathieu, L., and Budinger, T. F. (1974): Pinhole digital tomography. *Proceedings of the First World Congress of Nuclear Medicine*, pp.1264–1266. Japan.
16. Vogel, R. A., Kirch, D., LeFree, M., and Steele, P. (1978): A new method of multiplanar emission tomography using a seven pinhole collimator and an Anger scintillation camera. *J. Nucl. Med.*, 19:648.
17. Rogers, W. L., Brady, T. J., Koral, K. F., Keyes, J. W., Jr., and Thrall, J. H. (1979): Feasibility of tomographic gated blood pool imaging. *J. Nucl. Med.*, 20:628 (Abstract).
18. Kuhl, D. E., Abass, A., Reivich, M., Edwards, R. Q., Fenton, C. A., and Zimmerman, R. A. (1975): Computerized emission transaxial tomography and determination of local brain function. In: *Noninvasive Brain Imaging*, edited by H. J. DeBlanc, Jr. and J. A. Sorenson, p. 67. Society of Nuclear Medicine, New York.

19. Budinger, T. F., Gullberg, G. T., and Huesman, R. H. (1979): Emission computed tomography. In: *Image Reconstruction from Projections*. Vol. 32. *Topics in Applied Physics*, edited by G. T. Herman, pp. 147–246. Springer-Verlag, Berlin.

20. Gullberg, G. T. (1979): The attenuated Radon transform: Theory and application in medicine and biology. Ph. D. Thesis, University of California, Berkeley.

21. Chang, L. T. (1978): A method for attenuation correction in radionuclide computed tomography. *IEEE Trans. Nucl. Sci.*, NS-25(1):638.

22. Brownell, G. L., Correia, J. A., and Zamenhof, R. G. (1978): *Positron Instrumentation*. Vol. 5. *Recent Advances in Nuclear Medicine*, edited by J. H. Lawrence and T. F. Budinger, p.1. Grune and Stratton, New York.

23. Rankowitz, S., Robertson, J. S., Higinbotham, W. A., and Rosenblum, M. J. (1962): Positron scanner for locating brain tumors. *IRE Int. Conv. Rec.*, 10(9):49.

24. Ter-Pogossian, M. M., Phelps, M. E., Hoffman, E. J., and Mullani, N. A. (1975): A positron-emission transaxial tomograph for nuclear imaging (PETT). *Radiology*, 114:89.

25. Hoffman, E. J., Phelps, M. E., Mullani, M. A., Higgins, C. S., and Ter-Pogossian, M. M. (1976): Design and performance characteristics of a whole-body positron transaxial tomograph. *J. Nucl. Med.*, 17:493.

26. Cho, Z. H., Cohen, M. B., Singh, M., Eriksson, L., Chan, J., MacDonald, N., and Spolter, L. (1977): Performance and evaluation of the circular ring transverse axial positron camera (CRTAPC). *IEEE Trans. Nucl. Sci.*, NS-24(1):532.

27. Bohm, C., Eriksson, L., Bergstrom, M., Litton, J., Sundman, R., and Singh, M. (1978): A computer assisted ringdetector positron camera system for reconstruction tomography of the brain. *IEEE Trans. Nucl. Sci.*, NS-25(1):624.

28. Yamamoto, Y. L., Thompson, C. J., Myer, E., Robertson, J. S., and Feindel, W. (1977): Dynamic positron emission tomography for study of cerebral hemodynamics in a cross-section of the head using positron-emitting ^{68}Ga-EDTA and ^{77}Kr. *J. Computer Assist. Tomogr.*, 1:43.

29. Derenzo, S. E., Budinger, T. F., Cahoon, J. L., Greenberg, W. L., Huesman, R. H., and Vuletich, T. (1979): The Donner 280-crystal high resolution positron tomograph. *IEEE Trans. Nucl. Sci.*, NS-26(2):2790.

30. Muehllehner, F., Atkins, F., and Harper, P. V. (1977): *Positron Camera With Longitudinal and Transverse Tomographic Ability*. Vol. 1. *Medical Radionuclide Imaging*, pp. 291-307. IAEA, Vienna.

31. Lim, C. B., Chu, D., Kaufman, L., Perez-Mendez, V., Hattner, R., and Price, D. C. (1975): Initial characterization of a multiwire proportional chamber positron camera. *IEEE Trans. Nucl. Sci.*, NS-22(1):388.

32. Ter-Pogossian, M. M., Mullani, N. A., Hood, J. T., Higgins, C. S., and Currie, C. M. (1978): A multislice positron emission computed tomograph (PETT IV) yielding transverse and longitudinal images. *Radiology*, 128:477.

33. Ter-Pogossian, M. M., Mullani, N. A., Hood, J. T., Higgins, C. S., and Ficke, D. C. (1978): Design considerations for a positron emission transverse tomograph (PETT V) for imaging of the brain. *J. Computer Assist. Tomogr.*, 2:539.

34. Derenzo, S. E., and Vuletich, T. (1978): Scintillation performance of bismuth germanate crystals at low temperatures. Lawrence Berkeley Laboratory Report #7466, University of California, June.

35. Derenzo, S. E. (1979): Precision measurement of annihilation point spread distributions for medically important positron emitters. *Proceedings of the 5th International Conference on Positron Annihilation*, pp. 819-823. Japan.

36. Budinger, T. F., Derenzo, S. E., Gullberg, G. T., and Huesman, R. H. (1979): Trends and prospects for circular ring positron cameras. *IEEE Trans. Nucl. Sci.*, NS-26(2):2742.

37. Brooks, R. A., Sank, V. J., Talbert, A. J., and DiChiro, G. (1979): Sampling requirements and detector motion for positron emission tomography. *IEEE Trans. Nucl. Sci.*, NS-26(2):2760.

38. Mullani, N. A., Ter-Pogossian, M. M., Higgins, C. S., Hood, J. T., and Ficke, D. C. (1979): Engineering aspects of PETT V. *IEEE Trans. Nucl. Sci.*, NS-26(2):2703.

39. Derenzo, S. E. (1979): Optimization of side shielding for circular positron emission tomographs. Lawrence Berkeley Laboratory Report #9584, University of California, October.

40. Brownell, G., Burnham, C., Correia, J., Chesler, D., Ackerman, R., and Tavares, J. (1979): Transverse section imaging with the MGH positron camera. *IEEE Trans. Nucl. Sci.*, NS-26(2):2698.

41. Phelps, M. E., Hoffman, E. J., Huang, S.-C., and Kuhl, D. E. (1979): Design considerations in positron computed tomography (PCT). *IEEE Trans. Nucl. Sci.*, NS-26(2):2746.

42. Yano, Y., Budinger, T. F., Chiang, G., O'Brien, H. A., and Grant, P. M. (1979): Evaluation and application of alumina-based Rb-82 generators charged with high levels of Sr-82/85. *J. Nucl. Med.*, 20:961.
43. Budinger, T. F. (1979): Physiology and physics of nuclear cardiology. In: *Nuclear Cardiology. Cardiovascular Clinics*, edited by J. T. Willerson, pp. 9-78. Davis & Co., Philadelphia.
44. Smith, R. O., Love, W. D., Lehan, P. H., and Hellems, H. K. (1972): Delayed coronary blood flow detected by computer analysis of serial scans. *Am. Heart J.*, 84:670.
45. Fazio, F. M., Nardina, M., Fieschi, C., and Forli, C. (1977): Assessment of regional cerebral blood flow by continuous carotid infusion of krypton-81m. *J. Nucl. Med.*, 18:962.
46. Subramanyam, R., Alpert, N. M., Hoop, B., Jr., Brownell, G. L., and Taveras, J. M. (1978): A model for regional cerebral oxygen distribution during continuous inhalation of $^{15}O_2$, $C^{15}O$, and $C^{15}O_2$. *J. Nucl. Med.*, 19:48.
47. Welch, M. J., Thakur, M. L., Coleman, R. E., Patel, M., Siegel, B. A., and Ter-Pogossian, M. M. (1977): Gallium-68 labeled red cells and platelets: New agents for positron tomography. *J. Nucl. Med.*, 18:558.
48. Price, D. C., Hartmeyer, J. A., Prager, R. J., and Lipton, M. J. (1980): Evaluation of in vivo thrombus formation in dogs, using Indium-111-oxide labeled autologous platelets. In: *Indium-111 labeled neutrophils, platelets, and lymphocytes*, edited by M. L. Thakur and A. Gottschalk, pp. 183–186. Trivirum, New York.
49. Budinger, T. F., Yano, Y., Derenzo, S. E., Huesman, R. H., Cahoon, J. L., Moyer, B. R., Greenberg, W. L., O'Brien, H. A., Jr. (1979): Myocardial uptake of rubidium-82 using positron emission tomography. *J. Nucl. Med.*, 20:603 (Abstract).
50. Gould, L., Schelbert, H., Phelps, M., and Hoffman, E. (1978): Identification of 47% diameter coronary stenosis by noninvasive computed tomography of $^{13}NH_4^+$ during dipyridamole coronary vasodilation. *Circulation*, 58:11.
51. Hoffman, E. J., Phelps, M. E., Weiss, E. S., Welch, M. J., Coleman, R. E., Sobel, B. E., and Ter-Pogossian, M. M. (1977): Transaxial tomographic imaging of canine myocardium with ^{11}C-palmitic acid. *J. Nucl Med.*, 18:57.
52. Weiss, E. S., Hoffman, E. J., Phelps, M. E., Welch, M. J., Henry, P. D., Ter-Pogossian, M. M., and Sobel, B. E. (1976): External detection and visualization of myocardial ischemia with ^{11}C-substrates *in vivo* and *in vitro*. *Circ. Res.*, 39:24.
53. Ter-Pogossian, M. M., Weiss, E. S., Coleman, R. E., and Sobel, B. E. (1976): Computed tomography of the heart. *Am. J. Roentgenol.*, 127:79.
54. Brownell, G. L., Cochavi, S., Elmaleh, D. R., and Athanasoulis, C. A. (1979): Transverse section perfusion imaging in peripheral disease. *J. Nucl. Med.*, 20:619 (Abstract).
55. Tsui, E., and Budinger, T. F. (1978): Transverse section imaging of mean clearance time. *Phys. Med. Biol.*, 23:644.

*Noninvasive Techniques for Assessment of
Atherosclerosis in Peripheral, Carotid, and
Coronary Arteries*, edited by Thomas F.
Budinger, et al. Raven Press, New York
1982.

Commentary

K. Lance Gould

*Department of Medicine, University of Washington, Seattle Veterans Administration
Hospital, Seattle, Washington 98105*

Dr. Mock has asked us to describe methods for identifying plaques in the peripheral arteries. We can identify plaques fairly well using ultrasound, angiography, and some computerized angiographic methods. Advances are needed in application of the concepts, and some details need to be defined.

I call these techniques border contrast methods or shadow methods. We are looking at shadows and interfaces. We cannot image coronary plaques in the heart. Neither ultrasound, DSA, nor subtraction fluoroscopy with intravenous contrast media will identify coronary disease reliability.

That statement will probably bring a great deal of reaction, but I shall explain. The reason that I say this is partly theoretical. There is [inadequate] spatial and contrast resolution in all of these methods. They are compromises. In DSA, for example, temporal resolution is gained at the sacrifice of both spatial and density resolution.

I make this statement because when I look at coronary stenoses using the ultimate method, invasive, selective coronary arteriography, I get good results. However, if I try to quantify those lesions, I can just barely define the physiologic effects in terms of the pressure and flow changes. For example, if I want to measure the gradient in the flow in chronically stenosed animals, I first make an X-ray, then, using Brown's computerized quantitative technique, predict the pressure gradient. Compared with real-time imaging, even the best of cine X-rays are of borderline quality, even though in X-rays the temporal, spatial, and density resolutions are maximized.

Therefore, we cannot just choose a secondary method involving a sacrifice of resolution, saying that we are going to produce high-quality images with it. I think that the state of the physics will not allow it. Let me give you some specifics on why these methods do not work.

First, the pressure flow characteristics of stenosis in the coronaries are determined by fractions of a millimeter. In order to define any change affecting the patient or the physiologic animal, you must measure stenosis dimensions down to this level.

Second, stenoses are very dynamic. They have a life of their own. The normal artery varies in diameter, and the stenosis itself varies in diameter, and they vary independently of what is going on on the arterial bed. They are integrated differently, in a very complex interplay. The secondary branches, unlike the proximal coronary, may increase 100% in diameter. Furthermore, in high-flow states, when the pressure distal to the stenosis falls, the dimensions of the stenosis may change. This has been well documented in experiments soon to be published.

Finally, in the flexible stenoses arterial walls may collapse. At that point of such turbulence, the pressure gradient may change from 30 to 60 almost instantaneously, with no corresponding change in geometry whatsoever.

The presence of turbulence, with which the fluid engineers really have not yet come to grips, complicates the attempt to describe changes in the anatomic geometry. This means that we cardiologists are seeing shadows and borders, both in X-ray and ultrasound. Unless we take physiologic effects into account, we are going to miss a great deal. It is time for cardiology to go beyond shadows and look at the consequences in terms of metabolism and flow.

One answer to Dr. Mock's question of what these techniques can tell us about atherosclerotic plaques in the vascular system is that intravenous digital X-ray and ultrasound techniques will not work in the heart. If that statement can be proved wrong, this volume will have been of great benefit to us all.

We are up against an enormous physiologic problem if we must define the plaque in terms of shadows.

What are we left with?

The big question to me in cardiology is: Can we identify the lesions and make them regress with 99% certainty? The second question is: Is the cell alive or is it dead, or where in between is it?

The first question may be best answered by looking at flow distribution, not at the plaque, because I think the problems of noninvasive resolution of the plaque are prohibitive.

I think we can detect fairly minor lesions using positrons and good flow measurements. Even using first-generation equipment, we can detect 50% blockage. I am sure that we can detect down to 30 or 40% obstruction right now.

Whether the cell is alive or dead is a biologic problem that we do not yet know how to answer. I have not found a biochemist who will say at what point the cell dies. Whether cell death occurs when fatty acid metabolism stops or when glucose metabolism stops, related to membrane transport or myocardial function, is not clear. Positron imaging will likely allow us to measure the biochemical concentrations and determine whether the cell is alive or dead.

The two big questions may then be answered: Can you find the coronary lesion early, and is the myocardial cell alive?

Noninvasive Techniques for Assessment of Atherosclerosis in Peripheral, Carotid, and Coronary Arteries, edited by Thomas F. Budinger, et al. Raven Press, New York 1982.

Nuclear Detection of Atherosclerosis

H. William Strauss

Nuclear Medicine Division, Massachusetts General Hospital, Boston, Massachusetts 02114

The four approaches to the nuclear detection of atherosclerosis are: (1) measurement of lumen diameter, (2) local metabolism, (3) flow differential, and (4) changes in the permeability of the vessel wall. None of these methods is specific for the detection of an atheromatous plaque, but they can identify sites of arterial narrowing, measure flow differential distal to a hemodynamically significant lesion, and detect changes in local metabolism or permeability due to acute arterial injury. Such injury usually results in platelet and fibrinogen deposition at the injured site. Based on this knowledge, Thakur et al. (1) successfully identified damaged arteries with platelets labeled with an indium-111 oxine complex.

Finklestein et al. (2) have since determined the number of platelets required for a lesion to be visible on scan. First, they induced arterial lesions in rabbits by inflating a balloon in the distal aortas. Labeled platelets were then administered intravenously, followed by imaging 4 to 6 hr later. The animals were sacrificed, and their aortas were evaluated via scanning electron microscopy. Those animals showing lesions evidenced confluent layers of platelets at least two to three cells thick on the injured arterial wall.

Recent work by Khaw et al. (3), using technetium-labeled fibrinogen, indicates that this radiotracer also can identify sites of acute arterial and capillary injury. This may be accomplished using either labeled platelets or fibrinogen.

Another way to assess the impact of a hemodynamically significant obstruction on the distal pattern of perfusion is by nuclear angiographic examination. Rapid sequence images of the distribution of nuclides are recorded in the arterial and arteriocapillary phases after intravenous injection. Because the number of photons recordable during any one frame is limited by the dosage limit and rapid nuclide transit through the organ, only flow abnormalities greater than 50% can be reliably detected using this technique.

The methodology just described is too insensitive for general application using today's radiopharmaceuticals. Treves et al. (4), however, recently developed a more practical, ultra-short-lived iridium-191m tracer that permits doses up to 100 mCi. This gives a much greater photon yield and should permit higher-resolution images and thus improved lesion detection when using nuclear methods.

An alternative way to identify zones of abnormal flow distal to hemodynamically significant lesions utilizes tracers that follow the Sapirstein principle. Thallium-201, in the form of ionic thallous chloride, is most commonly employed (5); however, nitrogen-13, rubidium-82 (6) or water labeled with oxygen-15 (7) could easily be substituted. Intravenous thallium, rubidium or ammonia or inhaled carbon dioxide (which is converted to water in the lungs) will reveal systemic blood flow. In patients with significant narrowing of the iliac vessels, distribution of these tracers in the lower extremity of the involved side will usually be diminished (8). Thus, although the specific site of arterial disease cannot be identified by scanning, the extent of distal flow reduction can be seen. In the myocardium, furthermore, zones of diminished blood flow can be readily identified on the scan (9), although the specific coronary artery or arteries causing the abnormality cannot be readily identified.

Even with these limitations, thallium-201 has proved extremely useful in the detection of occult coronary artery disease. This method has a sensitivity of over 84% in tests using more than 1,800 patients (10).

Several techniques may be used to increase the contrast sensitivity of thallium imaging, including planar tomography (11) and transverse section tomography (12). Even using tomography, however, identification of flow disparities may remain difficult. Other abnormalities seen on the scan, such as zones of myocardial thinning, or increased lung uptake may serve as additional markers of coronary artery disease (13).

Another indirect way to identify zones of coronary artery narrowing is to evaluate cardiac function at rest and during exercise using either the first-pass or the equilibrium radionuclide technique (14). Although not specific for coronary artery narrowing (cardiomyopathies or valvular disease may also result in a decreased ejection fraction at exercise), the approach is extremely useful in screening. Concomitant measurement of changes in relative pulmonary blood volume (15,16) has been used to supplement the rest-and-exercise blood pool technique in the detection of occult ventricular dysfunction.

Several plaque-specific labeling techniques are under development. One involves the feeding of fats labeled with nonradioactive oxygen-18 to animals over a period of time, allowing their gradual assimilation by plaques. After the soft tissues having quicker cell turnover rates have cleared the labeled fat, an irradiating source "activates" the oxygen-18 to fluorine-18, which is detectable using a positron camera (17).

Lees et al. (18) have developed an iodinated lipoprotein radiopharmaceutical that enters the arterial wall of vessels undergoing intimal repair. These agents may serve to identify the atheromatous plaque directly.

Castronovo et al. (19) recently developed a long-lived phosphonate, labeled with iodine-125, specifically targeted to areas of calcium deposition. The long half-life of this radiopharmaceutical has allowed them to scan patients days to weeks after soft tissue clearance and identify arterial sites of calcium deposition.

Tracer procedures can successfully define the hemodynamically significant lesion. It is likely that a combination of such techniques will one day be used to detect the metabolic activity of atheromatous plaques.

REFERENCES

1. Thakur, M. L., Welch, M. J., Joist, J. H. et al. (1976): Indium-111 labeled platelets: Studies on preparation and evaluation of *in vitro* and *in vivo* functions. *Thromb. Res.*, 9:345.
2. Finklestein, S., Miller, A., Callahan, R., Godley, R., Fallon, J. T., Strauss, H. W., and Lees, R. S.: Imaging of acute arterial injury with Indium-111 labeled platelets—Comparison with scanning electron micrographs.
3. Khaw, B., Fallon, J., Strauss, H. W., Callahan, R., Covalo, A., and Haber, E.: A new method of labeling macromolecules with technetium-99m at neutral pH: Labeling anti-cardiac myosin and fibrinogen. *J. Nucl. Med. (in press).*
4. Hnatowich, D., Kulprathipanja, S., and Treves, S. (1977): An improved ^{191}Os-^{191}mIr generator for radionuclide angiocardiography. *Radiology*, 123:189.
5. Strauss, H. W., Harrison, K., Langan, J. K. et al. (1975): Thallium-201 for myocardial imaging—Relation of thallium-201 to regional myocardial perfusion. *Circulation*, 41:641.
6. Budinger, T. F., Yano, Y., and Hoop, B. (1980): A comparison of rubidium-82 and ^{13}NH$_3$ for myocardial positron scintigraphy. *J. Nucl. Med.*, 16:429.
7. Ackerman, R. H., Subramanian, R., Correia, J. et al. (1980): Positron imaging of cerebral blood flow during continuous inhalation of C^{15}O$_2$. *Stroke*, 11:45.
8. Christenson, J. T., Eklof, B., Hegedus, V., Jakobsson, A., and Westling, H. (1976): Examination of patients with ischemic vascular disease in the legs: What it is, what it should be. *Lakartidningen*, 73:2493.
9. Bailey, I., Griffith, L. S. C., Rouleau, J. et al. (1977): Thallium-201 myocardial perfusion imaging at rest and during exercise: Comparative sensitivity to electrocardiography in coronary artery disease. *Circulation*, 55:79.
10. Okada, R. D., Boucher, C. A., Strauss, H. W., and Pohost, G. M. (1980): Exercise radionuclide imaging approaches to coronary artery disease. *Am. J. Cardiol.*, 46:1188–1204.
11. Vogel, R. A., Kirsch, D., LeFree, et al. (1978): A new method of multiplanar emission tomography using a seven pinhole collimator and an Anger scintillation camera. *J. Nucl. Med.*, 19:648.
12. Treves, S., Holman, B. L., and Neirinck, R. (1979): Cardiac imaging with tantulum-178. *Radiology*, 131:525.
13. Barac, C., McKusick, K. A., and Strauss, A. W. (1982): Principles and techniques of cardiac nuclear imaging. In: *Cardiac Ultrasound and Nuclear Medicine*, edited by J. Morganroth and G. Pohost. *(in press).*
14. Borer, J. S., Kent, K. M., Bachrach, S. L. et al. (1979): Sensitivity, specificity and predictive accuracy of radionuclide cineangiography during exercise in patients with coronary artery disease. Comparison with exercise electrocardiography. *Circulation*, 60:572.
15. Okada, R. D., Pohost, G. M., Kirshenbaum, H. D., Kushner, F. G., Boucher, C. A., Block, P. C., and Strauss, H. W. (1979): Radionuclide-determined change in pulmonary blood volume with exercise: Improved sensitivity of multigated blood pool scanning in detecting coronary artery disease. *N. Engl. J. Med.*, 301:569.
16. Nichols, A. B., Strauss, H. W., Moore, R. M. et al. (1979): Acute changes in cardiopulmonary blood volume during upright exercise stress testing in patients with coronary heart disease. *Circulation*, 60:520.
17. Budinger, T. F.: Suggestion made during discussion session at the symposium on which this volume is based.
18. Lees, R., Lees, A., and Strauss, A. W. (1982): Extra corporeal imaging of human atherosclerosis. *Clin. Res. (Abstract)*, 30:398A.
19. Castronovo, F. P., Strauss, H. W., and McKusick, K. A. (1980): Radioiodinated phosphonic acid: A new agent for the study of bone resorption. *Soc. Nucl. Med., (abstract).*

Noninvasive Techniques for Assessment of Atherosclerosis in Peripheral, Carotid, and Coronary Arteries, edited by Thomas F. Budinger, et al. Raven Press, New York 1982.

Ultrasound Image Synthesis and Reconstruction

James F. Greenleaf, Lowell D. Harris, and Titus C. Evans, Jr.

Mayo Foundation, Mayo Medical School, Rochester, Minnesota 55901

Over the past 5 years, a high-resolution ultrasound imaging instrument has been developed and fabricated by Mayo-SRI (1). This instrument operates in a B-scan mode using 10 MHz pulsed ultrasound with an axial resolution of approximately 0.3 mm and a lateral resolution of approximately 0.6 mm. In most patients, B-scans can be obtained from 2 to 3 cm above to 5 to 6 cm below the carotid artery bifurcation.

It has become clear over the past 3 years, while scanning 300 patients using this model (2,3), that comprehension of the complete three-dimensional (3-D) character of the carotid artery and associated individual plaques and lesions is very difficult when using large sets of separate two-dimensional (2-D) B-scans of contiguous sections. Comprehension of a complex 3-D structure using sequential 2-D slices through that structure is especially difficult when certain aspects of the object to be imaged, such as a plaque, are not always visible, either because of spectral reflections of ultrasonic energy or because of high attenuation from overlying structures.

This problem is very similar to that experienced with X-ray CAT scan images. Reprojection imaging of 3-D CAT scan data has been shown to surmount successfully such problems (4). For this reason, we have developed techniques for constructing complete, 3-D ultrasound images of the carotid artery and its lesions using computerized methods of perspective projection (5).

Sets of parallel B-scans are obtained by digitizing the video output of the scanner at a 5 megasample/sec rate. A sequence of parallel transaxial scans covering a 2.7 cm segment of the bifurcation of the excised human carotid artery are then stored on digital magnetic tape. These individual 2-D images (Fig. 1) are then stacked in a 3-D array in the memory of the computer and displayed by projecting the volume pixel elements (voxels) of the image array onto a plane. This produces the 2-D image array, which is suitable for display on a television monitor. The computer forms these arrays called projection images, by mathematically summing the magnitude of the voxels along selected parallel (line of sight) paths through the volumes of data for isometric displays and along converging paths for perspective images.

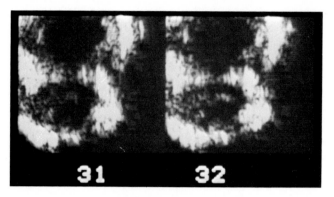

FIG. 1.   Examples of two (numbers 31 and 32) of the 64 B-scans used to construct a 3-D array of brightness values that were stereoptically projected onto viewing planes (see Fig. 2).

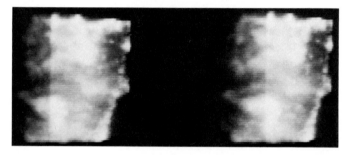

FIG. 2.   Stereoptic views of a volume of data consisting of 64 sequential digitized B-scans obtained from a digitized, *in vitro* carotid artery. Volume was "sliced" along the lumen of the artery and data nearest the viewer were discarded, allowing an unobscured view of the character of the far wall of the artery. A 3-D effect may be obtained by viewing the left image with the right eye and the right image with the left eye.

Also being evaluated are the techniques of numerical "dissolution" and "dissection," whereby portions of the display volume that obscure regions of interest are either partially dissolved or totally eliminated prior to projection (4,5). These methods allow complete regions of the volume of data to be discarded or analyzed separately.

A 3-D projection of a set of B-scans from an *in vitro* carotid artery is shown in Fig. 2. The volume of data was cut in half, with the plane of sectioning through the midline of the common carotid and the internal and external carotid arteries. The "front" half was removed, and the coronal section nearest the viewer (which slices through the center of the lumen of the common, internal, and external carotid arteries) was "brightened." The volume was then mathematically rotated by 6° and reprojected to obtain the stereoptic pair of views shown in Fig. 2. By crossing one's eyes, i.e., looking at the left image with the right eye and the right image with the left eye, one can see the 3-D character of this carotid artery. On the far wall of the carotid artery is a region of ultrasound scatter, which may be due to a plaque in the arterial wall but was not caused by a large lesion.

The use of this technique *in vivo* seems straightforward. Sequences of B-scans, as in Fig. 1, can be obtained at incremental lengths along the artery at a rate of up to 20/sec, and—with or without synchronization of the image with the heart rate—it is probable that useful, 3-D ultrasonic images of the carotid artery can be constructed. A prime advantage of this technique is that the volume images can be sliced down the lumen of the artery and two halves of the volume can be viewed separately, as though the observer were actually inside the lumen.

The addition of parametric surfaces representing Doppler velocities within the lumen would be an additional advantage and, combined with the 3-D B-scans, should permit quicker and fuller evaluation of the character of the lumen than would be possible using individual, 2-D cross-sectional images of the lumen. The data further suggest that a few 3-D images of the lumen, perhaps one for each view (the anterior and posterior views), would provide a complete record of the lesion, thus obviating the necessity of keeping the results of 2-D B-scans in the patient's record.

REFERENCES

1. Evans, T. C., Green, P. S., and Greenleaf, J. F. (1974): Mayo Foundation Report No. NO1-HT 42904-1.
2. Mercier, L. A., Greenleaf, J. F., Evans, T. C., Sandok, B. A., and Hattery, R. R. (1978): High-resolution ultrasound arteriography: A comparison with carotid angiography. In: *Noninvasive Diagnostic Techniques in Vascular Disease*, p. 231. C. V. Mosby, St. Louis.
3. Greenleaf, J. F., Kottke, B. A., and Evans, T. C. (1977): Early diagnosis and detection of atherosclerosis. In: *Atherosclerosis Reviews* (2), p.187. Raven Press, New York.
4. Harris, L. D., Robb, R. A., Yuen, T. S., and Ritman, E. L. (1979): Display and visualization of three-dimensional reconstructed anatomic morphology: Experience with the thorax, heart, and coronary vasculature of dogs. *J. Computer Assist. Tomogr.*, 3:439.
5. Harris, L. D., Greenleaf, J. F., and Evans, T. C. (1979): Display of 3-D ultrasonic images. *Acoustical Imaging*, 9:227.

Noninvasive Techniques for Assessment of
Atherosclerosis in Peripheral, Carotid, and
Coronary Arteries, edited by Thomas F.
Budinger, et al. Raven Press, New York
1982.

Correlation of Noninvasive Methods with Angiography: Carotid Arteries

Paul M. Chikos, Jack H. Hirsch, Lloyd Fisher, Brian L. Thiele, and D. E. Strandness, Jr.

Department of Surgery, University of Washington School of Medicine, Seattle, Washington 98195

In attempting to validate the accuracy of noninvasive tests for the detection of carotid artery disease, the only standard for comparison is contrast arteriography. These X-ray studies are best when multiple views are taken, with selective injection of the contrast material into the common carotid arteries. This procedure, when well performed, provides as good a resolution as can be obtained in nearly any area of the circulation. There is little doubt that such studies can help determine normalcy or the presence of disease with a high degree of accuracy. Since the arteriogram directly measures the internal dimensions of the artery, it should be possible theoretically to make accurate measurements of the degree of plaque involvement in terms of diameter reduction, as well as of the nature of surface changes, whether smooth, irregular, or ulcerated.

Most diagnostic tests can be classified as indirect or direct. Indirect tests for arteriosclerosis detect disease by measuring changes in pressure and/or flow at some point distal to the bifurcation, such as the ophthalmic artery, the first branch of the internal carotid artery. Direct tests derive information from the carotid bifurcation itself, either by imaging or by measuring disturbances in flow caused by atherosclerotic plaquing.

Indirect tests are considered positive when the available collateral pathways that bypass the carotid bulb are called into play. This point is presumably reached when the stenosis becomes severe enough to reduce pressure and flow. The indirect test will thus remain positive, unless some therapeutic maneuver is carried out that either restores carotid blood flow to normal or markedly improves it.

Direct testing theoretically could provide information about the condition of the carotid bulb at all stages of arteriosclerosis. Thus, if such tests are made sufficiently sensitive, they should not only predict the degree of narrowing, but also provide baseline studies for following the natural history of the disease. In practice, however, it is necessary to compare the early results of the noninvasive tests with those obtained using contrast arteriography. This approach presumes, of course, that the contrast studies are sufficiently accurate to provide this essential comparison.

191

In the initial stages of our validation studies, we established a grading scheme as the working basis for the subsequent comparisons. We defined five separate arteriographic categories by degree of stenosis as follows: normal, $< 10\%$ (defined as wall roughening alone), 10 to 49%, 50 to 99%, and total occlusion. It quickly became apparent that we needed to establish the inter- and intraobserver variability in reading the arteriograms, both in terms of the five categories and in estimating the degree of diameter reduction of the common, internal, and external carotid arteries.

To evaluate our performance, tests of 128 carotid arteries with four views of the internal carotid were reviewed by three radiologists in two separate readings. The tests were randomly assigned and read at a rate of 16 cases/week for 8 weeks. All lesions were measured using calipers; normal diameter was estimated to the nearest 0.5 mm and degree of stenosis to the nearest 5%.

We will consider only the data from our internal carotid tests. First, the question of intraobserver variability between two readings, as determined for each of the three observers: The absolute difference in their estimation of residual diameter ranged from 5.98 to 6.29%, with the average being $6.04 \pm 8.09\%$ [1 standard deviation (SD)]. The correlation coefficient was 0.98 ($N = 384$). When the five angiographic categories were compared, complete agreement as to the grouping was noted in 83.3% of the arteries.

When interobserver variability was examined, similar rates were found. The average difference in degree of stenosis measured was $8.64 \pm 9.50\%$ (1 SD). The correlation coefficient among readers was 0.98 ($N = 1,536$). Across the five angiographic categories, there was agreement in 75% of the arteries measured. Redefinition of the second and third as 1 to 24% and 25 to 49% did not improve the accuracy of this separation.

When the data were plotted in increments of 5% (using 0 as normal and 100% as total occlusion), comparison of both intra- and interobserver measurements revealed considerable scatter. For each reading of the intraobserver studies, there was agreement within 5% in only 41.4% of the arteries studied. When the interobserver variability was reviewed in a similar fashion, there was agreement in 30.1% of the readings.

Even the difference in choice of angiographic category in classifying the arteries was not insignificant, ranging from 17 to 25%. The extent of the variability is most evident in the lesser stenoses, where small differences in readings often determined the category of placement. Further interpretive problems are caused by the asymmetry of the plaque, as seen in the human—the degree of stenosis observed in one plane may not equal that observed in another view.

While it remains to be shown, it is unlikely that ultrasonic imaging will prove more accurate than angiography in grading lesions. When flow disturbances are considered the hallmark of disease, they apparently can be related with reasonable accuracy to the broad categories of angiographic involvement that we used. Further, it is likely that measurement of velocity disturbances at exactly the same location in each examination will provide the most sensitive method of documenting atherosclerotic progression.

Noninvasive Techniques for Assessment of Atherosclerosis in Peripheral, Carotid, and Coronary Arteries, edited by Thomas F. Budinger, et al. Raven Press, New York 1982.

Validation of Performance in the Examination of Peripheral and Coronary Arteries

Donald W. Crawford and Robert H. Selzer

Department of Cardiology, University of Southern California, Los Angeles, California 90033; and Biomedical Image Processing Laboratory, Jet Propulsion Laboratory, California Institute of Technology, Pasadena, California 91109

If angiography is to be used as an indirect measure of some of the characteristics of atherosclerosis, or as validation for the performing of noninvasive methods, accuracy must be examined. To do this, one must first consider the goal of the study. Distinguishing surgically significant stenosis from no stenosis in an artery 5 mm in diameter and detecting a 250 μm thickness change in a nonobstructive lesion for a regression trial are considerably different tasks. We review here our experience with the validation of several angiographic methods for the examination of peripheral and coronary arteries. This work has resulted from the collaboration of several co-investigators, in particular, Drs. David H. Blankenhorn, Samuel H. Brooks, and Robert Barndt, Jr.

Clearly, one of the necessary approaches in validation of performance for the detection of atherosclerosis is correlation with a direct measure of pathology. Most angiographic-pathologic correlations have been limited to study of obstructive disease, excluding thinner, less complex lesions. However, for regression trials, a safe method for the examination of less than obstructive lesions is clearly desirable. We studied this approach in a peripheral (femoral) artery in particular.

Femoral angiograms were made in cadavers under simulated clinical conditions using a pressurized radiopaque casting material (1). After dissection, arterial segments were matched and coded with reference to the permanent casts. The opened arterial segments were sequenced by four graders in increasing order of disease on the basis of the International Atherosclerosis Project grading scheme. The segments were then assayed for cholesterol.

The angiograms from the cadavers were subject to image dissection and computer analysis, using various computer indices of edge irregularity chosen as likely candidates for comparative quantification of atherosclerosis. Of 13 indices correlating significantly with visual grade and cholesterol, two predicted visual grade, and three, cholesterol content.

A simplified computer estimate of atherosclerosis (CEA), using one computer-derived variable, has resulted from this work and has been used to examine the error involved in the computerized estimate of atherosclerosis and atherosclerotic change (2). Using a combination of radiographic phantoms, cadaver casts, and studies of serial films exposed in the same sequence from single clinical angiograms, we estimate the coefficient of variation of a single determination is 6% (of a 1 to 128 score), when conditions are ideal, to 14%, when conditions are adverse, depending on a range of factors including body habitus, amount of injected contrast, and changing radiographic technique. Therefore, an estimate of the upper limits of CEA error might better be obtained directly from clinical angiograms.

Estimation was approached as follows: 32 patients with premature myocardial infarction had three sequential angiograms suitable for CEA analysis (3). We assessed error by using the simplifying assumption that atherosclerotic change is a linear process. Linear least squares equations were written for each individual to furnish 112 estimates of CEA error. The average error was 6%; for a segment in the middle range of atherosclerosis, the coefficient of variation approached 18%. Since this estimate includes all pooled factors, we consider it an upper limit.

Certain conceptual difficulties arise when using a pathologic measure of atherosclerosis to calibrate a digitized angiographic method that is naturally quantitative. A comparison of the first with the second or third assessment is not a function of grades derived from pathology, and it is difficult to give an arbitrary pathologic order to the complex lesions, such as hemorrhagic ulcers and stenosis. In addition, several stages of disease of possible clinical significance may be present in a small region. Therefore, we visually graded segments of cadaver specimens according to the exemplary, homogeneous classes of normal, stenotic, and hemorrhagic ulcer (4) and compared them with available position postmortem angiograms.

Computer-derived measurements used in this examination were the ratio of minimum width to average width, as well as various edge roughness indices. Of 27 exemplary lesions, 26 were classified correctly by the jackknife procedure.

Another conceptual difficulty arises from both the use of visual grading of pathologic specimens and the use of computer-derived measurements based on edge roughness or indentation. No measure of atherosclerosis in satisfying physical units of true area or volume can be derived. In an attempt to overcome this, we modified the angiographic densitometric equations of Hilal so that chord lengths of contrast medium across a vessel contour could be derived from single plane angiograms using quantitative densitometry (5). Summation of cross-sectional chord length is an estimate of cross-sectional area; summation of areas over increments in length yields volume. In cadaver angiograms of diseased vessels using arterial cast slices for comparison, areas derived from cadaver films were highly correlated (r = 0.997) with those measured from the cross-sectional slices. Accuracy of chord length measurement was ±0.28 mm in vessels 4 to 10 mm in diameter. The confidence limits for measurement of enface plaque were 14% by area for 5 mm diameter arteries and 6% for 8 mm arteries. The method is now being applied to larger scale computerized studies.

Another index can be derived from quantitative densitometry. It is a common observation that arteries in life are regular or smooth, not only by edge longitudinally—but also in cross section, where the regularity is essentially circular. Given a cross-sectional diameter, a mathematical index of regularity is easily derived. It can be shown that a function of angiographic optical densities is exactly proportional to this mathematical index of regularity if the vessel is perfectly circular or elliptical in cross section (4). Deviations from proportionality are indices of atherosclerosis on a very local level.

Against the background of evaluation of femoral atherosclerosis summarized previously, we proceeded to evaluate experimental angiograms in dogs. In this study, the selective angiogram has been the reference against which is compared relatively noninvasive first pass venous angiography (6). Intravenous contrast delivery removes some of the risk of arterial tree invasion but provides images with less information individually. We obtained useful images (carotid) by computer averaging of films exposed during the first pass from a peripheral vein in large dogs given 25 ml Renografin-76. Six films obtained in rapid sequence were digitized and 15 cm sections of carotid were studied.

In a typical case, selective arteriogram scatter of adjacent discerned edge points was 46 μm, while single venous film edge scatter was 94 μm. Composites of six venous injection films with two-dimensional image smoothing reduced scatter to 31 μm. Thus, in these normal vessels, the uncertainty of edge location in single or multiple composite venous injection images could be compared to the demonstrably more precise selective arteriograms. Similar approaches may be applicable to studies of diseased vessels.

The study of the coronary arteries, even by angiography, is more difficult, but approachable. As compared with many peripheral arteries, the coronaries are highly mobile and tortuous. We have developed programs to track the edges of arbitrarily curved coronary arteries and to produce a computer-generated lumen (7). We believe it likely that computer-generated quantitative densitometry calculations of cross-sectional area, regularity, and segmental volume can be applied to these vessels with reference to previous quantitative experience with peripheral arteries. Our initial experience would suggest that the major origins of both coronaries can be visualized and computer analyzed, using various first pass angiograms. It appears critically important to be able to analyze the first portions of the coronary tree by semi-invasive or noninvasive means; if significant coronary atherosclerosis is present, it is present in these locations. We believe this can be done, and our current work in first pass venous angiography has this goal.

REFERENCES

1. Crawford, D. W., Brooks, S. H., Selzer, R. H., Barndt, R., Jr., Beckenbach, E. S. and Blankenhorn, D. H. (1977): Computer densitometry for angiographic assessment of arterial cholesterol content and gross pathology in human atherosclerosis. *J. Lab. Clin. Med.*, 89:378.
2. Blankenhorn, D. H. (1978): Quantitative angiography. In: *Very Early Recognition of Coronary Heart Disease*, edited by L. McDonald, J. Goodwin, and L. Resnekov, pp. 27–42. Intl. Congress Series 435. Excerpta Medica, Amsterdam-Oxford.

3. Blankenhorn, D. H. (1978): Quantitation of atherosclerosis in peripheral blood vessels. *Intl. Conference on Atherosclerosis*, edited by L. A. Carlson et al., pp. 417–422. Raven Press, New York.
4. Brooks, S. H., Crawford, D. W., Selzer, R. H., Blankenhorn, D. H., and Barndt, R., Jr. (1978): Discrimination of human arterial pathology by computer processing of angiograms for serial assessment of atherosclerosis change. *Comput. Biomed. Res.*, 11:469.
5. Crawford, D. W., Brooks, S. H., Barndt, R., Jr., and Blankenhorn, D. H. (1977): Measurement of atherosclerotic luminal irregularity and obstruction by radiographic densitometry. *Invest. Radiol.*, 12:307.
6. Selzer, R. H., Crawford, D. W., Brooks, S. H., and Blankenhorn, D. H. (1979): Synthesis of carotid arteriograms by intravenous contrast delivery and multiframe computer averaging. *Circulation*, 60:11 *(Abstract)*.
7. Selzer, R. H., Blankenhorn, Crawford, D. W., Brooks, S. H., Barndt, R., Jr. (1976): Computer analysis of cardiovascular imagery. *CALTECH/JPL Conference on Image Processing Technology, Data Sources and Software for Commercial and Scientific Applications*, pp. 6–20. November. Pasadena, Calif.

Noninvasive Techniques for Assessment of Atherosclerosis in Peripheral, Carotid, and Coronary Arteries, edited by Thomas F. Budinger, et al. Raven Press, New York 1982.

Validation Studies of a Noninvasive Real Time B-Scan Imaging System

M. Gene Bond, Ward A. Riley, *Ralph W. Barnes, Janet M. Kaduck, and Marshall R. Ball

*Bowman Gray School of Medicine, Wake Forest University, Winston-Salem, North Carolina 27103; and *Department of Surgery, Medical College of Virginia, Virginia Commonwealth University, Richmond, Virginia 23298*

In order to be of diagnostic value in evaluating atherosclerosis, noninvasive ultrasound instruments that produce arterial images must accurately reflect the state of the artery, i.e., the images produced must be valid, reliable, and reproducible. As with all noninvasive techniques, the images produced should be compared to and correlated with accepted invasive standards, such as images produced by X-ray, but also, when possible, with the gross specimens of the arteries.

The purpose of this chapter is to describe the *in vitro* method we are using to validate a 5 MHz real time B-scan imaging system and to compare and correlate B-scan images, derived from human common carotid arteries obtained at autopsy, with radiographs, as well as with the gross and microscopic specimens.

METHODS

Segments of common carotid arteries, measuring 7 cm in length, were obtained from human cadavers at autopsy. The artery was visualized *in situ* and a line drawn along the anterior midline for orientation of the specimen during evaluation. Three sites from each artery were chosen at 1.0 cm intervals for interrogation and were marked by circumferential lines drawn on the adventitial surface. The artery was removed, flushed briefly with normal saline to remove postmortem blood clots, mounted horizontally in a heated water bath, and oriented with the anterior midline facing up. The artery was then cannulated and perfused with saline at a standard pressure (100 ± 5 mm Hg).

Constant pressures during the imaging were maintained by using calibrated manometers and regulator valves. The mounting apparatus allowed for rotation of the artery at 1° increments through an arc of 360°. The anterior midline was designated 0°. The ultrasound beam was aligned directly over each of the three sites to be examined using a laser. The interaction of ultrasound with the laser allowed positioning of the beam over the sites to be examined with an accuracy of approximately

±0.5 mm. To assure that the ultrasound was incident perpendicular to the normal axis of the vessel to within ±1°, careful angle adjustments of the ultrasound beam were performed to maximize the light-sound interaction. The artery was then rotated, with the ultrasound transducer remaining stationary, to each of the four angles of interrogation, 0°, +45°, −45°, and +90°. Individual photographs were taken at each angle and lumen diameter and wall thickness measured from each photograph.

Arteries were interrogated using a 5 MHz linear array ultrasound system, designed and constructed at the Bowman Gray School of Medicine at Wake Forest University. The transducer array consisted of 32 rectangular elements, 3.8 mm in length × 0.64 mm in width and spaced by intervals of 0.15 mm. A line of image information was obtained by exciting five adjacent elements of the array in phase during the transmit operation and summing reflected signals from seven elements during the receive operation. The signals from individual elements were logarithmically amplified prior to summing. A total of 23 image lines, spaced approximately 0.8 mm apart, were obtained in this manner as groups of elements were electronically scanned at a 10 Hz rate. An image frame rate of approximately 400 Hz resulted from this excitation. The field of view formed by the image was approximately 5 cm in depth and 2 cm in width. The axial and lateral resolution of this system was measured in a water tank by observing the echo reflected from a point metal reflector located 15 mm from the transducer face. The lateral resolution measured, using the −6 dB points of the video signal, was 1.1 mm. The corresponding axial resolution was approximately 0.4 mm.

Calibration was accomplished by using dimensional markers spaced at known intervals on the photograph and assumed an average sound speed in tissue of 1,540 m/sec. A correction factor was used to adjust measurements prior to data analysis to account for the small differences between sound velocity in soft tissue and water.

After B-scan interrogation, the vessels were pressure-perfusion-fixed in the heated water bath with 10% neutral buffered formalin (100 ± 5 mm Hg). At the end of 3 hr of fixation, each artery was perfused with barium gel/sulfate mass (100 ± 5 mm Hg). The artery was then radiographed at 0°, +45°, −45°, and 90° directly on an X-ray cassette (Du Pont Cronex 4 film with par speed screens) with a 40 inch focus to film distance using a 0.3 mm focal spot tube (1/20 sec, 50 MA, 50 KVP). Dimensional markers were placed adjacent to the artery at each site being examined and X-rayed with each specimen for calibration purposes. The resolution of this system was measured at 7 line pairs/mm. Measurements of lumen diameter were made from X-ray films using a magnified micrometer reticle graduated in 0.1 mm intervals and then corrected for calibration.

After X-ray, the artery was transected perpendicular to the longitudinal axis at each of the three sites, and measurements were made of lumen diameter and arterial wall thickness at each angle. Care was taken to ensure that measurements made from the radiographs were compared to the corresponding measurements obtained from the B-scans and gross specimens. This is important since the basic process of image formation using X-rays is fundamentally different from that of the B-scan.

RESULTS AND DISCUSSION

The range in arterial lumen diameters obtained from the gross specimens used in this study was approximately 5.0 to 7.5 mm. Although severe atherosclerotic lesions, as measured by lumen stenosis, were not present in any specimen, all arteries did have some degree of lumen narrowing, which ranged from 1 to 9%.

Average lumen diameter measurements determined from B-scan images, radiographs, and gross specimens are presented in Table 1. Average lumen diameter measurements determined from B-scan cross-sectional images and radiographs compared well with measurements made from the gross specimens. Overall, there was a tendency for the measurements of lumen diameter determined from B-scan images to be slightly larger, however, than those measured from the gross specimens. When comparing data points derived from these two methods, there also tended to be an increase in the absolute differences, especially in arteries where the lumen diameter was less than 5.5 mm (Fig. 1).

Average lumen diameter measurements made from radiographs were slightly underestimated when compared with the gross specimens; however, the mean absolute difference between gross and X-ray measurements (0.3 ± 0.2 mm, mean ± SD) was smaller than between the gross and B-scan measurements (0.5 ± 0.1 mm). There was also an increase in the absolute difference between gross and X-ray measurements in arteries where the lumen diameter was less than 6.5 mm (Fig. 2).

The range in arterial wall thickness measured from gross specimens was approximately 0.6 to 1.8 mm. The mean arterial wall thickness and correlation coefficient derived from B-scan images and gross specimens are presented in Table 2.

The majority of arterial wall thickness measurements made from B-scan images were larger than those from the corresponding gross specimens. The mean absolute difference between the two methods was 0.6 ± 0.3 mm. Unlike measurements of lumen diameter comparing the two methods, the variability in difference between B-scan and gross measurements of arterial wall thickness was approximately the same regardless of the size of the artery wall (Fig. 3).

Correlation coefficients were used to compare the variability and predictability in estimating lumen diameter and wall thickness. Measurements made from radiographs, when compared to the gross specimens, showed less variability in absolute

TABLE 1. *Comparisons of lumen diameter*

	Gross (mm)	X-ray (mm)	B-scan
Mean ± SD	6.1 ± 0.5	5.9 ± 0.4	6.2 ± 0.5

Correlation coefficients		
Gross vs. X-ray	r = 0.76	(N = 147 pairs)
Gross vs. B-scan	r = 0.42	(N = 132 pairs)
X-ray vs. B-scan	r = 0.33	(N = 132 pairs)

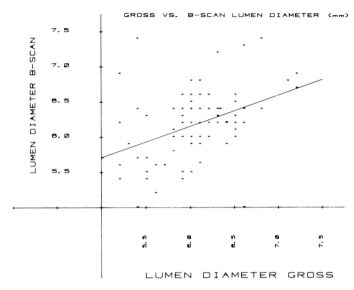

FIG. 1. Linear regression of lumen diameters (mm) obtained from gross specimens and B-scan images.

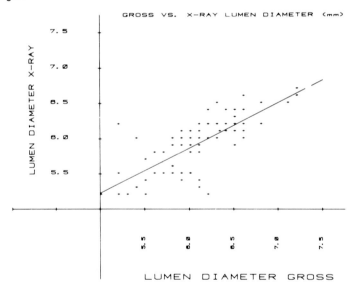

FIG. 2. Linear regression of lumen diameters (mm) obtained from gross specimens and radiographs.

differences between the two methods (r = 0.76) and were more predictive of the gross specimens than were those made from B-scan images (r = 0.42). Analysis of radiographic measurements with B-scan measurements resulted in a correlation coefficient of 0.33. Arterial wall thickness measurements determined from B-scan

TABLE 2. *Comparison of arterial wall thickness*

	Gross (mm)	B-scan
Mean ± SD	1.0 ± 0.2	1.3 ± 0.4
Correlation coefficient		
Gross vs. B-scan r = 0.30	(N = 132 pairs)	

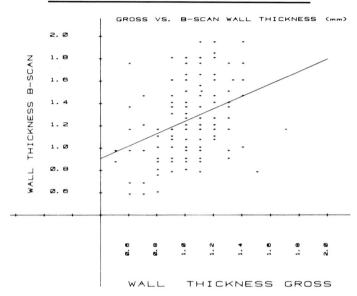

FIG. 3. Linear regression of arterial wall thickness (mm) obtained from gross specimens and B-scan images.

image were also compared to the gross observation and resulted in a correlation coefficient of 0.30.

Although we were unable to visualize the entire cross-sectional surface of the majority of arteries using real time B-scan imaging *in vitro*, we attempted to determine if it was feasible to estimate the minimal amount of atherosclerosis present in these vessels from the image obtained. From each site we had four independent B-scan images of lumen diameter at angles of 0°, +45°, −45°, and 90° relative to the anterior midline. We assumed that the largest lumen diameter was present in that orientation of the artery that had the least amount of atherosclerosis. That, in fact, was a reasonable assumption, based on both grand microscopic sections of the relatively few sites of arteries we have examined thus far using this method (eight of 42 sites). Using this diameter measurement and assuming that the lumen contour of a normal human common carotid artery is approximately circular, we mathematically calculated the maximum lumen area. To determine the percentage of lumen stenosis, we averaged all four lumen diameters from a given site, calculated the area within the circle described by the average diameter, and expressed the results as a ratio ($\times$ 100) of the maximum lumen area.

The assumptions made in these calculations may not be valid for segments of arteries that are not circular, e.g., bifurcations, nor for arteries in which athero-sclerotic lesions are symmetrically circumferential (stenosis would be underesti-mated), nor in cases in which severe stenosis is present (stenosis would also be underestimated in this case). For this study, however, the minimal intimal changes observed were not symmetrical, and the contour of the innermost elastic lamina was very close to being circular. The same method used to evaluate B-scan images was also used to estimate the percentage of lumen stenosis from radiographs. The actual percentage of lumen stenosis was determined from microscopic sections (Verhoeff-Van Gieson stain) by measuring the length of the innermost elastic lamina and by calculating the area from this circumference. Lumen area was measured and calculated in a similar manner. Microscopically, lesions were present in each of the arteries studied ($\bar{x}$% stenosis, 5.8; frequency of stenosis, 8/8; range, 2 to 9%). Similar determinations from radiographs were $\bar{x}$% stenosis, 2.5; frequency of stenosis, 7/8; range, 0 to 5%; and from B-scan images, $\bar{x}$% stenosis, 12.5%; frequency of stenosis, 8/8; and range, 5 to 20%. The observed microscopic values from percent lumen stenosis from microscopic sections was 2 to 9%. Measurements from radi-ographs and B-scan images correctly identified 6/8 (75%) and 3/8 (38%) of the cases within this range, respectively.

We would like to emphasize the point that we were not able to estimate the percentage of lumen stenosis by visual estimation from any single B-scan image or radiograph, but that we were able to discern relatively subtle differences by applying morphometric techniques to both methods of evaluation.

The lesions observed microscopically in eight of the 42 sites being examined were composed of smooth muscle and fibroblast-like cells, collagen, ground sub-stances, and fine elastic fibrils. In general, these lesions contained diffuse accu-mulations of interstitial, oil red O, stainable lipid. In no case did we observe in our B-scan evaluations of these relatively thin lesions, tissue characteristics that differentiated the lesion from the underlying tunica media.

SUMMARY

In this preliminary report we have described our methods for validating a 5 MHz real time B-scan imaging system using excised segments of human common carotid arteries obtained at autopsy. Measurements of lumen diameter, wall thickness, and percentage of lumen stenosis, determined under fairly rigid experimental conditions, were made from B-scan images, radiographs, and gross and microscopic specimens of arteries.

Our findings suggest that there is close agreement between average lumen di-ameters measured from B-scan images, radiographs, and gross specimens, but that there is also more variability in attempting to predict wall thickness from B-scan images. The correlation coefficient found when comparing B-scan images to gross specimens was 0.42 for lumen diameter and 0.30 for wall thickness and clearly reflects this unexplained variability. Considering the relatively small size of these arteries and the resolution of the 5 MHz system being evaluated, there are several potential artifactual or interpretive errors that may explain part of this variability, including interrogation of the artery at slightly different orientations during B-scan imaging, interpretive errors in determining the position of the intimal-lumen interface, artifacts caused by fixation or temperature changes, or slight pressure differences during perfusion fixation.

The ultrasound measurements were obtained from the unprocessed B-scan image, which is limited by the range resolution. With additional signal processing, such as wall thickness determination by spectral analysis methods, a higher degree of accuracy can be obtained. As a result, we should expect the correlation coefficients to improve significantly.

In conclusion, we suggest that the findings of this *in vitro* study cannot be extrapolated directly to either the *in vivo* condition, nor, in general, to other ultrasound systems that have not been validated morphologically. We would hope, however, that similar studies would soon be initiated at other laboratories to expand considerably the scope of knowledge in this area and to help assess the quantitative limits of the various medical imaging modalities.

Noninvasive Techniques for Assessment of Atherosclerosis in Peripheral, Carotid, and Coronary Arteries, edited by Thomas F. Budinger, et al. Raven Press, New York 1982.

Methods of Morphologic Assessment of Coronary Atherosclerosis Pertaining to Noninvasive Techniques

A. S. Daoud, J. Jarmolych, K. E. Fritz, and W. A. Thomas

Albany Medical Center, Albany, New York 12208

For noninvasive techniques for assessment of coronary atherosclerosis to be of any clinical value, the results should correlate well with the anatomical findings in these vessels. As a basis of such correlation, an accurate, objective, and practical method is needed for morphologically quantitating the arterial disease. A number of methods—gross (1–4), microscopic (5,6), and/or biochemical (7,8)—have been described for assessing coronary atherosclerosis. The gross evaluation of coronary atherosclerosis is made on cross sectioned or longitudinally opened arteries.

In general, since noninvasive techniques rely on coronary blood flow and/or on arterial lumen size, the use of longitudinally opened arteries for evaluation is not suitable for correlation with these procedures. Biochemical methods are also not suitable for this purpose because the information as to lumen and lesion size is sacrificed during the procedure.

We have developed methods suitable for comparing results of examinations by noninvasive techniques with morphologic findings in the coronary arteries. In the past, we have used these methods in assessing human atherosclerosis in geographic and epidemiologic studies. At present, we are in the process of modifying them to be used in an experimental study of progression and regression of atherosclerotic lesions in swine, where coronary angiography assessment is paralled with detailed morphologic studies. This study is being carried out with members of the Cardiology Department of the University of Massachusetts at Worcester. The modified methods that are projected to be used in examination of swine hearts can easily be applied to human hearts.

GROSS EVALUATION OF CORONARY ATHEROSCLEROSIS

The heart is removed with a portion of the ascending aorta. The coronary arteries are perfused with saline and injected with a radio-opaque substance and angiographed. After angiography, the coronary arteries are then perfused with a 10% formaldehyde solution and fixed for several hours. The components of the heart,

205

with particular emphasis on the myocardium, are examined for fresh or healed infarction or focal fibrosis. If infarction is present, it is charted on a special form. This form provides a schematic diagram of the myocardium, divided and subdivided, so that the observer may locate precisely the anatomic site of the infarcts and their relationship to branches of the coronary arteries. The size and stage of the infarct are also noted on the chart.

The coronary arteries are cut at 5 mm intervals. Every segment is examined for the presence or absence of atherosclerotic plaques. If present, the type of plaque (fatty or fibrous) is noted. Also noted is the presence of calcification, hemorrhage in plaque, or thrombosis. The lumen and the thickness of the wall of every segment are measured by specially designed calipers made specifically for this purpose. They are composed of two separately movable jaws with a movable post held in position between the jaws. With this instrument, simultaneous measurements of the lumen and of the arterial wall can be made.

The method is reproducible, and wall thickness is found to correlate well with the presence of myocardial infarction (9).

MICROSCOPIC ASSESSMENT OF CORONARY ATHEROSCLEROSIS

A description of the method used in our laboratory follows. The coronary arteries are cross sectioned at 5 mm intervals and the segments are fixed in formalin and embedded in carbowax. Four consecutive sections are taken from each block and stained with the following stains: hematoxylin and eosin, oil red 0 for lipids, Verhoeff-Van Gieson for fibrous and elastic tissue, and iron stains for blood products.

Quantitation of atherosclerosis can be done in several ways. One way is to calculate the mean lumen diameter and mean wall and intimal thicknesses. Using an ocular micrometer and Verhoeff-Van Gieson stained sections, the mean luminal diameter of each segment is calculated by averaging the greatest and smallest diameters of the lumen. The mean intimal and wall thicknesses are calculated in a similar manner. In another approach, the lumen area, the intimal area, and the entire arterial wall area can be measured by counting squares of an ocular grid. More recently, a system for quantitative digital image analysis is being used. Using the same techniques with various special stains, the areas occupied by necrosis, fat, calcium deposit, etc. can be calculated in each individual lesion. Quantitative digital image analysis is particularly suitable for this purpose.

COMMENT

In the assessment of coronary atherosclerosis in the living patient, the most important aspect is the volume flow/unit of time through the artery. Clearly, most of the postmortem pathologic methods discussed are not designed to provide direct information on flow through the vessel during life. It is very likely that a close relationship exists between the amount of coronary atherosclerosis as measured by these methods and the rate of flow during life, since a direct relationship between myocardial infarction and the amount of atherosclerosis has been reported by several investigators using the various techniques. Figure 1, a bar graph from our data, compares by decade the mean coronary wall thickness (MCWT) of 194 men with, and 482 without, myocardial infarcts. It is apparent that those with myocardial infarcts have much greater MCWT at any age than the corresponding individuals without infarct. It is also apparent, in the group without myocardial infarcts, that the MCWT increases progressively with age, while it does not change appreciably with age in the infarcted group. Similar findings were noted in females. While the morphologic methods cannot correct for postmortem changes per se, the close correlation of the amount of the disease found in the coronary arteries at postmortem examination and the evidence of ischemic heart disease indicates that these alterations, if they occur, are of minimal significance (9).

The gross methods of assessing coronary atherosclerosis are based on the premise that coronary wall thickening is a fair index of the degree of atherosclerosis. In our opinion, except for rare instances, this assumption seems justified since (a) in general, atherosclerosis causes thickening of coronary arterial walls through the accumulation of such abnormal substances as lipid, fibrous tissue, calcium, and products of hemorrhage, and (b) except in rare instances, appreciable thickening of coronary arterial walls is due only to atherosclerosis and its complications.

Irregularity of the lumen of markedly diseased arteries poses the problem as to which diameter one should measure. Some measure the smallest diameter while others use the mean of the largest and smallest diameters. We have chosen to

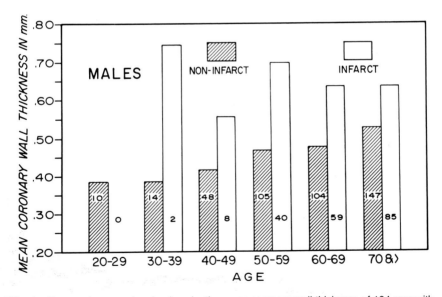

FIG. 1. Bar graph comparing, by decade, the mean coronary wall thickness of 194 men with, and 482 men without, myocardial infarcts. It is apparent that those with myocardial infarcts have much greater MCWT at any age than the corresponding individuals without infarct. It is also apparent that in the group without myocardial infarcts, the MCWT increases progressively with age.

measure the diameter in the plane parallel to the epicardial surface. It is also critical to determine the intervals along the course of the arteries at which measurements should be made. In a special study, we measured the coronary arteries at 1 mm through 1 cm intervals and found that mean coronary wall thickness and mean lumen size are approximately the same if measurements are based on segments 1 through 5 mm in thickness. The microscopic methods also have their own pitfalls.

These are alterations due to fixation and embedding, malorientation of the sections, and sampling. The changes due to processing are probably constant for all segments and likely to have little effect on the overall evaluation of the disease. Indeed, a good correlation between the amount of disease, as estimated microscopically, and the presence of ischemic heart disease has been demonstrated in virtually all studies reported. The orientation of the segment requires extreme care that all sections are cut perpendicular to the axis of the artery. As to sampling, the same criteria discussed in the gross methods probably apply to the microscopic techniques.

In conclusion, there is no perfect method for absolute quantitation of coronary atherosclerosis. However, gross and microscopic methods, adequate for the purpose of correlation of noninvasive techniques with morphologic findings, exist. The microscopic methods are preferable because of the wider spectrum of variables that can be relatively quantitated.

REFERENCES

1. Daoud, A. S., Goodale, F., Florentin, R., and Beadenkopf, W. G. (1962): Chemicoanatomic studies in geographic pathology. *Arch. Pathol.*, 73:74.
2. Holman, R. L., McGill, H. C., Jr., Strong, J. P., and Geer, J. C. (1958): The natural history of atherosclerosis: The early aortic lesions as seen in New Orleans in the middle of the 20th century. *Am. J. Pathol.*, 34:209.
3. Ackerman, R. F., Dry, T. J., and Edwards, J. E. (1950): Relationship of various factors to the degree of coronary atherosclerosis in women. *Circulation*, 1:1345.
4. White, N. K., Edwards, J. E., and Dry, T. J. (1950): The relationship of degree of coronary atherosclerosis with age, in men. *Circulation*, 1:645.
5. Scott, R. F., Daoud, A. S., Wortman, B., Morrison, E. S., and Jarmolych, J. (1966): Proliferation and necrosis in coronary and cerebral arteries. *J. Athero. Res.*, 6:499.
6. Young, W., Gofman, J. W., Malamud, N., Simon, A., and Waters, E. S. G. (1956): The interrelationship between cerebral and coronary atherosclerosis. *Geriatrics*, 11:413.
7. Fritz, K. E., Augustyn, J. M., Jarmolych, J., Daoud, A. S., and Lee, K. T. (1976): Regression of advanced atherosclerosis in swine. *Arch. Pathol. Lab. Med.*, 100:380.
8. Augustyn, J. M., Fritz, K. E., Daoud, A. S., Jarmolych, J., and Lee, K. T. (1978): Biochemical effects of moderate diet and clofibrate on swine atherosclerosis. *Arch. Pathol. Lab. Med.*, 102:294.
9. Daoud, A. S., Florentin, R. A., and Goodale, F. (1964): Diffuse coronary arteriosclerosis versus isolated plaques in the etiology of myocardial infarction. *Am. J. Cardiol.*, 14:69.

Noninvasive Techniques for Assessment of Atherosclerosis in Peripheral, Carotid, and Coronary Arteries, edited by Thomas F. Budinger, et al. Raven Press, New York 1982.

Commentary

Jesse E. Edwards

Department of Pathology, United Hospitals, St. Paul, Minnesota 55102

This volume was designed to consider the nature of atherosclerosis, and the various ways of measuring it and of identifying its stages. In so doing, we should not assume that there is any bottom line in coronary atherosclerosis but disability and death. Also, we should not oversimplify the problem by thinking that the worse the atherosclerosis gets, the worse the patient's corpse is.

While we do accept that there is such an entity as atherosclerotic coronary disease, its various clinical manifestations have not correlated very well with the observed degrees of change. For example, in measuring the degree of coronary atherosclerosis in patients with various levels of stable and unstable angina, one finds no significant correlation between them. There is even some question about the use of the word "degree"—How accurately are we measuring? Even according to various accepted definitions of degree, we cannot see any difference in the amount of atherosclerosis from one test to another.

Another very disturbing problem is sudden death in coronary disease, which is probably the number one cause of death in the United States. In the overwhelming majority of patients who die suddenly from coronary atherosclerosis, the pathology of the coronary system does not reveal any acute change indicating why yesterday an individual seemed to be perfectly healthy but today he is dead.

Obviously, the problem of coronary atherosclerosis has many aspects besides assessment. We cannot see such things as spasm in the diseased segments or in the collateral system.

For example, an individual has severe obstructive disease in the anterior descending coronary artery without infarction. At the same time, the lumen of the anterior descending artery becomes so small at the site of greatest involvement that the distribution of blood to the myocardium is impaired. The patient then has a coronary thrombosis and develops an extensive myocardial infarction. If he was living on the collateral system because his lumen was so small, why did luminal thrombus cause the infarction?

Perhaps the underlying rupture of the plaque caused a hemorrhage or stimulated vasospasm in the collateral vessels that had been keeping the myocardium alive.

Noninvasive Techniques for Assessment of
Atherosclerosis in Peripheral, Carotid, and
Coronary Arteries, edited by Thomas F.
Budinger, et al. Raven Press, New York
1982.

Commentary

Clarence E. Davis

Department of Biostatistics, University of Washington, Seattle, Washington 98105

I am going to try to summarize from a statistical point of view what I see as the problems, and some solutions, of validating the procedures about which we have written. I also want to try to answer some of the questions that were raised.

If we were to plot the results of a standard test for measuring degree of atherosclerosis, which I will call X, against some other measuring procedure, which I will call Y, we might expect to get a straight line through the origin, indicating perfect agreement between the two tests. Invariably, however, when we estimate this slope, we do not get a straight line.

There are two potential reasons for this: There may not, in fact, be perfect agreement between the two procedures, and there is usually statistical variability in the measurement. If I estimate the slope with some variability in my standard measure, I underestimate the slope by a quantity $\sigma^2/(\sigma^2 + \sigma_m^2 + \sigma_s^2)$.

The quantity, σ^2, is the variability among my patient population. The quantity, σ_s^2, I will call short-term biological variability, and σ_m^2, is the variability among my measures, which include such things as intraobserver variability, problems associated with producing the images, etc.

The larger these two quantities are, the smaller the slope is going to be when plotted in this way. As you will recall, Dr. Dodge used a slide similar to this, and I believe this duplicates at least part of what he has seen.

While this formula presents part of the problem in statistical terms from my point of view, it also shows us some of the solutions and is a way of tying together the various procedures for validation that we have been talking about.

If I choose the diameter of a pipe as a standard, I eliminate one source of variability. That pipe should not change in diameter; thus it is better than whatever I am using to measure now. That would leave only measurement as a variable. This is not a very realistic solution for actual measurement, but it nonetheless gives us some information.

On the other hand, if I were to measure an autopsied artery as a potential standard, I suspect it would prove smaller than it was when alive. So there is some variability due to the procedure, yet we still include it in our measurement.

Now, I am still writing about the standard, not the new test.

Finally, when I actually do angiography, I may find a third variable: short-term physiologic changes in the individual. By "short-term," I mean within a few weeks or a few days.

Now, that seems to be the bad news, and it is my way of viewing the question of what we have been looking at. The good news is that I think, according to the studies presented by Drs. Bond, Strandness, and others, that we are beginning to delimit these variables or at least to recognize some determinants of their size.

As a statistician, if I have good, precise measurements of these components, I can adjust my estimates to bring this line of agreement closer to equality. If, after my adjustments, I still get a line with a slope less than 1, then I will say that perhaps the two tests do not, in fact, measure the same thing—and I think that this problem is compounded by the question of whether or not our various tests really are measuring the same thing. So, hopefully, we can agree on good ways of correcting for these errors.

My readjustment process is not a new way of describing the variables problem. It was first outlined in the 19th century; so we have known about it for a long time. We do not have good solutions for it. In the statistical literature, it is called "errors in variables" or "structural regression."

If I see a correlation between these two, rather than this regression situation, I find this term—actually, the square root of this term—and the square root of the same term for my new test multiplying that correlation. If I have a lot of measurement error problems in my standard and in my new test, I end up with a poor correlation. Therefore, I must, as best I can, reduce these sources of variability in my comparison of the standard and the test if I want a good correlation.

To comment specifically, Dr. Bond used some correlations that were quite small. As he pointed out to me in a conversation, part of the problem is that he was looking at the correlation in a restricted range. When I restrict the range, I will get a smaller correlation as well.

If I use a scatter diagram, I may get a very good correlation. But if I restrict my computation to a small range of data, the points begin to look more like a circle, and the correlation is smaller. I believe that is part of Dr. Bond's problem.

To Dr. Strandness, I have to say I was amazed that those correlations, inter- and intraobserver, were as high as they were. My results with cardiologists reading ECGs are not nearly as good, in most instances. Those look good to me, as opposed to being troublesome.

I have something to add to his question of why, when you categorize, things get a little worse. But before I get to that, I will say that his apology for categorization is interesting. Statisticians have the same arguments about whether to categorize the data or use a linear model, so you can probably find a statistician to meet with your clinical point of view.

This is another look at Dr. Strandness' example of intraobserver variability. For purposes of categorization, let us divide the data into quadrants, take 50, and across here at 50. We are only going to consider these two categories.

For the most part, the misclassified observations fall at, or near, the boundary.

The least squares procedure measures orthogonally down to this line and weighs in this average, and it says, "This point appears to be 55 and 50." If I cut off at 50, that point gets thrown in as a miscategorization. The least squares does not give much weight to that point, says it is not really very far off. Categorization, however, does. So, this is one partial explanation for what happens.

Now, here are four observations that are way off, no matter what you look at. The least squares method will include them, but you will notice, as Dr. Fisher pointed out, that you have 40 up here and 30 down here in this corner, plus quite a few on the diagonal. These things, when you average over the whole group, these four observations do not get much weight, so the correlation remains high. That is my attempt at a statistical explanation for what happened.

Now, in connection with what Drs. Daoud and Edwards mentioned about the autopsy and about the myocardial infarction (MI), I would like to raise a question.

I am involved in a Lipid Research Clinic, one of the large-scale trials sponsored by the National Heart, Lung, and Blood Institute. We have 4,000 men in this study, and we are taking 7 years to find out whether lowering cholesterol is going to prevent heart disease.

Our endpoint is MI. That is why we need so many years and so many men. We would be very pleased to do the study using 10% of those men over a 2-year period—if we had some way of measuring atherosclerosis. But our ability to measure atherosclerosis is not really direct, so our endpoints must be either myocardial infarction or sudden death.

My question then, given all this background, is: Would some of these noninvasive and more direct measures of atherosclerosis be appropriate for such studies were they begun today? That is what this volume is supposed to address, and I am putting it in personal terms.

Noninvasive Techniques for Assessment of
Atherosclerosis in Peripheral, Carotid, and
Coronary Arteries, edited by Thomas F.
Budinger, et al. Raven Press, New York
1982.

Commentary

Harold T. Dodge

*Department of Medicine, Division of Cardiology, University of Washington,
Seattle, Washington 98105*

My colleagues and I have been using techniques to quantify the arteriosclerotic, atherosclerotic lesions. We have been very interested in the problems of validation, and I will comment on some of our experiences.

First, I would like to comment briefly about our methodology.

The way we conduct our studies, the data on lesions are read by two or three technicians; they are all done in duplicate. It takes us months to train persons to do these studies. It is not the kind of thing you do casually—there is more skill and training involved than might appear at first.

We worked with Dr. Reichenbach, our pathologist, in developing the method for quantifying the atherosclerotic lesions in postmortem vessels. Initially, the vessels were injected with contrast medium, an opaque mass that solidifies in the vessels. These vessels were filmed, dissected, fixed, and cut into microscopic sections. The lumen was planimetered and the dimensions determined microscopically and then compared with the dimensions previously determined by X-rays of the dissected specimens. The agreement was ±80 μm.

Recently, we have tried to do the same thing in hearts that we reinjected prior to their being fixed. We have experienced a lot of problems with our method, and we have been working for a couple of years to solve them.

One problem is that the injectate often has little bubbles, which show up in the X-ray film. We have to work out a way to debubble the injectate.

Another problem occurs when you prepare the vessel for sectioning so that you can planimeter it to determine the dimension microscopically: The fixation process causes additional shrinkage of the tissue. We have not yet found a way to solve that problem.

That has been our experience with pathology to date. Validation using postmortem material is not easy.

There is one other way of characterizing lesions that has not been discussed. What you see in one plane on a film projection does not necessarily represent the entire length of the segment. But if you have two views, it is possible to compute the spatial characteristics of the segment and the actual length of the narrow segment. Then we can compute the values of the atheromatous mass, which is made up of the material that is projecting into the lumen between the two ends of the vessel segment. I am not sure if this is another useful way to characterize atheromatous lesions, but we make these calculations as part of our angiographic studies.

Finally, I would like to say something about our experiences with dimensions of lesions in patients who have different kinds of problems, because it gives us some additional perspective on what we are trying to do with instrumentation techniques.

The normal left anterior descending coronary artery lumen is about 3.2 to 3.5 mm in diameter. When disease is first recognized, the vessel lumen is about 1.5 mm in diameter.

In a group of patients who had had a syndrome of unstable angina without evidence of infarction, we found the diameter of the coronary artery supplying that region of the heart to be about 0.88 mm. But in patients who had had subendocardial infarction, the diameter was found to be about 0.64 mm.

The changes we have observed over the course of the disease or after drugs were given have been in the range of about 20%. Therefore, we need techniques that can detect changes in vessel diameter at the level of about 0.1 mm.

In patients who have local abnormalities, we have looked at the arterial segments supplying the portion of the ventricular wall where these abnormalities exist. Where the lesions are isolated, we do not see abnormalities, unless the cross-sectional area of the coronary artery is in the range of 0.5 mm squared or smaller. You must have good techniques to see these lesions and to quantify them as indicators of significant disease.

One of our procedures is to use the tip of the catheter as a standard of measurement comparison. We have been working with some of the catheter manufacturers to try to improve this technique. The tip of a No. 8 coronary catheter is about 2.72 mm and a No. 7 catheter is about 2.3 mm in diameter. It is nearly the size of the coronary artery, and it is very helpful to have this measuring scale right in the lumen. It would be even more helpful if the manufacturers would produce a catheter with a metallic tip on it or some device allowing one to see it a little better than a regular catheter tip.

Noninvasive Techniques for Assessment of Atherosclerosis in Peripheral, Carotid, and Coronary Arteries, edited by Thomas F. Budinger, et al. Raven Press, New York 1982.

Coronary Arteries

Thomas F. Budinger

Donner Laboratory University of California, Berkeley, California 94720

The charge to the coronary artery researchers in this volume stressed the need for noninvasive methods of detecting, measuring, and describing the coronary artery plaques that can also be used to follow the history of their size progression or regression and any changes in their chemical or structural composition. Such methods would help in the staging of patients who are good candidates for lumen dilation, in understanding the natural history of arterial disease, and in following any changes due to remedial therapy for coronary artery disease in a particular patient cohort. Three techniques approach these objectives: tissue composition characterization by multienergy or monoenergetic, photon-computed tomography, radionuclide imaging of the distribution and localization kinetics of radiopharmaceuticals likely to be specific for certain types of plaque tissue, and nuclear magnetic resonance measurements of arterial wall fat composition and flow.

Other techniques, although applicable in carotid and other peripheral arteries, were considered inadequate methods for plaque characterization because coronary arteries are relatively small, are attached to a heterogeneous reflecting surface, are rapidly moving targets, and are immersed in a large-volume, dynamic tissue system—the thorax.

However, the team did identify important alternate objectives for their deliberations, namely, the selection of methods to detect the presence of very early coronary artery disease in asymptomatic patients. The group agreed that, where invasive techniques must be used at some point in the staging of patients, an appropriate approach (at least for the research stage) would be to investigate the sensitivity of tissue signatures using 100 to 200 MHz ultrasound transducers on coronary vascular probes. *In situ* measurement of β and γ emitters that have attached to plaques is another possibility.

The consensus of the committee with regard to X-ray, ultrasound, nuclear magnetic resonance, microwave, and radionuclide imaging is presented below in that order.

X-RAY TECHNIQUES

The committee acknowledged that the gold standard—selective arteriography—most consistently reveals where and how large the lesions are. Measurement of vessel diameter changes, fixing of lesion position, and plaque size estimation are also possible using computerized arteriographic techniques. Small improvements can be expected in X-ray guns, but this will probably not change the course of diagnosis or increase the understanding of lesion pathophysiology. Lowered inter-observer variability rates and other improvements in selective arteriography can also be expected; however, arteriography tells us very little about the plaque and is not a noninvasive technique.

Digital Subtraction Angiography

In this volume, the technique of digital subtraction angiography (DSA) has been discussed, along with results of early DSA patient studies of the peripheral arteries made at the University of Wisconsin. Some researchers have begun imaging the coronary tree using this technique. The coronary artery working group agreed that there is sufficient promise in the intravenous angiography method (which uses two views to delineate the presence of disease in coronary arteries) that more research in this technique should be encouraged. The system at the University of Arizona has a spatial resolution expectation of 1 mm, with 0.5% contrast resolution. Data can be collected at 30 frames per sec for a raster of 512 × 512. With low doses and short patient imaging times (5 to 10 sec), one can expect to achieve a resolution of less than 0.5 mm, thanks to this system's new microfocal spot tube, which is capable of about 4 × 1 magnification. This intravenous contrast infusion technique for noninvasive imaging of coronary arteries needs to be further evaluated, with special attention to the following:

1. Although the dynamic range of state-of-the-art image intensifier-TV systems is adequate, poor signal-to-noise ratios due to quantum statistics might limit their ability to detect coronary arteries overlying ventricles filled with contrast medium. A contrast change of 1 mm in 30 mm can be expected, and a minimum contrast resolution of 0.5% should suffice. Image processing and the use of edge-detection algorithms should allow one to see the coronary tree using DSA, even when vessels overlie the ventricles.

2. Monoplanar DSA projections from different patients will show large variations in relationships of the coronary tree relative to the ventricular contrast; however, this might be solved by using two views that can vary in direction.

3. The problem of background motion has hampered users of digital subtraction methods. Motion around the heart gives a background variability that is not easily compensated for by breath-holding. The problem is not seen in high target-to-nontarget contrast arteriography; however, subtraction of images having a background mismatch of densities produces serious artifacts, which appear as contrast noise greater than expected when distinguishing arteries overlying ventricular contrast medium. More research is needed here.

Computer Tomography Tissue Chemistry Characterization

The recently marketed monoenergetic tube may emit nearly monoenergetic beams of sufficient intensity to allow differences in attenuation as a function of energy to be translated as tissue chemical composition. Its potential is great for distinguishing among plaques with lipid accumulation, plaques that are completely fibrous, and plaques having a given minimum atom percentage of calcium.

The technique requires two or three nearly monoenergetic beams, used to make a CT scan. As has been shown by other groups not represented in this volume but active in the field, the dosage is not prohibitive when multiple X-ray energies are produced using various filters with standard X-ray guns on conventional CT machines.

Monoenergetic scanning may prove a valuable means of determining the tissue class to which plaques belong, but further testing is needed. This technique should be evaluated along the following lines in order to better understand its feasibility and potential:

1. Theoretical CT imaging studies using state-of-the-art monoenergetic beams should be made, with varying spatial and atomic composition resolutions, and configurations. We need to know how well one can distinguish among coefficients reflecting differences in plaque composition within reasonable scan times of up to perhaps 30 min and radiation doses of less than 10 rads to the abdomen.

2. In order to understand the meaning of such changes in coefficients, it is important to observe the actual coefficient levels corresponding to important changes in the pathological and chemical composition of plaques of 1 to 2 mm in size.

3. The implementation of this approach in the human coronary tree requires rapid, volumetric imaging systems, such as the dynamic spatial reconstructor (DSR) at Mayo Clinic.

The Dynamic Spatial Reconstructor

The Mayo Clinic's new DSR instrumentation, intended for imaging epicardial and endocardial motion, is also able to image the coronary tree and show transmural perfusion. Though its resolution in coronary tree imaging is 1 to 2 mm, it can delineate overall anatomical configuration. This instrument has promise for both early diagnosis and sequential evaluation of the progression or regression of disease in individual patients.

ULTRASOUND

Current ultrasound technology is inadequate for imaging coronary artery plaques and for ascertaining tissue characteristics. Exceptions to this, along with specific limitations and suggestions for improvement, are as follows:

1. The need to penetrate the thorax with high frequencies limits one's use of swept frequencies and spectral analysis in tissue characterization, as is done in larger vessels,

such as peripheral arteries. There is a need for methods of using esophageally placed transducers and transcutaneous imaging with signal averaging and gating.

2. Ultrasound at present can see only 10% of the coronary tree. It can, however, reliably reveal lesions in the proximal 2 cm of the main coronary artery.

3. Ultrasound may be used to evaluate changes in the makeup of tissues, which we believe will include plaque changes. To do this, one might pass a catheter having an ultrasound transducer through the femoral artery into the abdominal and thoracic aorta, which will bring signal frequencies close enough to the tissues to allow such a tissue signature approach. This method might be useful in a study of the life course of plaques under various conditions in a group of patients.

More research is needed before the true potential of ultrasound in imaging the coronary arteries can be assessed.

NUCLEAR MAGNETIC RESONANCE

The working group believes that nuclear magnetic resonance (NMR) techniques have the potential to determine changes in tissue characteristics by measuring relaxation times and that they may also be useful in measuring flow. Their applications are, however, presently limited to the carotid and peripheral arteries. They might one day be used to image the coronary arteries, but with perhaps too poor a resolution (probably 2 to 3 mm) to be of great benefit, since these vessels move rapidly.

The aorta is also a good target for NMR studies using whole-body systems, which might allow one to examine relaxation times in tissue that can be stabilized using ECG gating. The results should prove much better than those resulting from examination of the coronary arteries.

The potential use of NMR imaging in biological research in conjunction with such markers as fluorine, phosphorus, or injected manganese was discussed by some of the working group, and it was generally agreed that these media are not promising for either the problem of plaque characterization or that of early coronary artery disease diagnosis in the asymptomatic patient due to low sensitivity.

MICROWAVE AND OTHER METHODS OF IMAGING

The state of the art in microwave imaging, as used by groups at Walter Reed Army Hospital, the University of Chicago, and elsewhere, was not reviewed in this volume. However, we noted the following:

1. Microwaves can be very sensitive detectors of the chemical composition and molecular arrangement of tissues.

2. The microwave scatter problem can potentially be solved using techniques well known to scientists dealing with the inverse problem.

3. Microwave's high capability in identifying molecular configuration is very poorly matched by the low imaging resolution of these long-wavelength photons.

An imaging system that can achieve the fine resolution necessary has yet to be demonstrated in theory or practice.

4. The electrical characteristics of tissues expressed as a bulk parameter, such as conductivity as a function of frequency, are very important to consider when searching for new methods for characterizing tissues, such as plaques, which change with time. Conductivity may change by factors of 10 from one region of the coronary artery to another, yet no method at present can measure these changes noninvasively.

EMISSION IMAGING AND EMISSION TOMOGRAPHY

Three applications of emission imaging have been discussed in this volume: functional recording of changes in ventricular cavity dimensions using labeled red cells or similar intravascular tracers, imaging of the myocardium with single photons or positron emitters in order to infer flow and metabolism, and imaging the distribution of tracers that might be specific to plaques or various types of tissues involved in the evolution of plaques. The first method is used in the analysis of symptomatic coronary artery disease. This is not a new approach, but it is still under development in the research community.

Thallium emission imaging has been shown to be a somewhat more sensitive detector of early coronary artery disease than ECG stress testing; however, its accuracy record is poor for coronary artery stenoses in the range of 50%, and it was thus not considered by the working group as sufficiently sensitive to warrant added research. Positron emission tomography, on the other hand, is a proved technique for measuring specific volume flow in tissue volumes as small as $2 \times 2 \times 1$ cc in the human myocardium and can detect human infarctions as small as 4 cc. In addition, it can measure aerobic and anaerobic metabolism and thus is a sensitive measure of the consequences of coronary artery disease. Using emission tomography with positrons (or, perhaps, with the proper instrumentation, single photons), one may evaluate patients before and after exercise or pharmacological intervention. This should reveal any hemodynamically significant lesion; however, exact localization and characterization of the flow-reducing plaque or distribution of plaques cannot be achieved by positron tomography myocardial imaging without special tracers specific for the plaque region.

PLAQUE TISSUE RADIONUCLIDE TAGS

As was demonstrated in 1976, it is possible to label platelets with gallium 68 or indium 111 and then to measure the accumulation of the labeled platelets on injured vessel walls. Over the past 2 years, researchers have demonstrated a limited potential of this method in measuring the distribution of platelets in man; however, problems in labeling and platelet injury during the labeling procedure have been overcome and some renewed activity might occur. The working group agreed that the specificity of this method has been high enough to warrant further studies of labeling as a technique for detecting thrombi and active embolization.

In addition to gallium- and indium-labeled platelets, labels that might prove specific for plaque tissues include: technetium 99m-labeled fibrinogen, iodine 123-labeled phospholipids, low-density lipoproteins labeled with iodine or some other appropriate radionuclide, acetate labeled with carbon 11, and labeled antibodies. Problem areas remaining in developing this technique include:

1. Anticipated low uptake kinetics of label in atheromata or plaques.
2. Low rate of clearance of the tracer from the blood pool and adjacent tissues.
3. Measurement of the specificity of label uptake in various types of arterial pathophysiology.
4. Establishment of the safety of antigen-antibody systems proposed for use in man.

We concluded that emission tomography techniques could prove useful in early detection of coronary artery disease and that the use of these techniques should be fostered to evaluate the efficacy of bypass surgery and medical intervention as therapeutic treatment for coronary artery disease.

Noninvasive Techniques for Assessment of Atherosclerosis in Peripheral, Carotid, and Coronary Arteries, edited by Thomas F. Budinger, et al. Raven Press, New York 1982.

Carotid and Iliofemoral Artery Imaging Systems[1]

James F. Toole and *Robert W. Barnes

*Department of Neurology, Bowman Gray School of Medicine, Wake Forest University, Winston-Salem, North Carolina 27103; and *Department of Surgery, Medical College of Virginia, Virginia Commonwealth University, Richmond, Virginia 23298*

CAROTID ARTERIES

Every year, nearly 600,000 people in the United States become stroke victims, most as the direct result of atherosclerosis. Approximately 40% of these die within a month, and at least two-thirds of those who survive have permanent disability. The population of the United States currently includes 2½ million disabled survivors of stroke.

With the aging of our population and the control of heart disease and cancer, the problem of stroke will take on increasing importance for health care and economic planners. Behavioral abnormalities secondary to cerebrovascular disease, including poststroke dementia, personality changes, mood and memory impairment, and loss of specific skills, will assume increasing importance and must be addressed.

It is estimated that about 70% of strokes are caused by atherosclerosis. Carotid artery disease is responsible for nearly half of all infarctions due to atherosclerosis and accounts for about 20% of all strokes. Over 90% of carotid plaques are found in patients with infarction due to carotid disease, about half of whom experience a transient ischemic attack (TIA) within a month prior to infarction. Regarding the two main possibilities, occlusion or embolism, as many as 60% of patients with carotid disease may have their stroke secondary to embolism from a carotid plaque. This group is likely to have warning TIAs.

The variety of definitions and methods used to collect and analyze data on TIAs has made it extremely difficult to get reliable information. The prevalence of TIAs,

---

[1]Author's note: Some material herein is excerpted from the report of the cerbrovascular disease panel of the Working Group on Arteriosclerosis, NHLBI, January 1979.

however, approaches 5/1,000/year in the population aged 65 years and over. The stroke risk for this segment is between 4 and 10 times that of the control population without TIAs and may reach 35% within a 4-year period. TIA is thus one of the best indicators of impending cerebral infarction. About 30% of patients with TIAs of the carotid artery have other clinically detectable signs of arteriosclerosis in the carotid arteries, such as murmur or abnormalities in the collateral circulation through the external carotid artery.

There is a pressing need to identify populations at high risk of myocardial infarction by applying acceptable, reliable, and cost-effective methods of detecting disease in the carotid arteries in the neck. In order to identify this group before infarction occurs, traditional techniques of history review and clinical examination must be employed, so that patients at high risk for cerebral circulatory insufficiency can be identified. This cannot be effected without appropriate educational programs for health care professionals. Patients with symptoms must have rapid and easy access to the health care system for detection of remediable disorders and prevention of stroke. At the present time, from 9 to 27% of patients with TIAs have normal angiographic evaluations. Furthermore, arteriography carries with it a major complication rate of about 2%. There is thus a great need to identify more precisely those patients in whom angiography is indicated. Because one-half of all TIA patients succumb to myocardial infarction within 5 years, there is also a need to develop means for identifying concomitant, asymptomatic arteriosclerotic plaques in the coronary arteries in order to reduce the high risk of myocardial infarction in TIA patients.

Ultrasound systems to detect lesions at the carotid bifurcation cannot meet the need to visualize the entire cerebral arterial tree. This includes both carotid arteries, both vertebral arteries, and their intracranial ramifications. Only when these four arteries and their collateral and anastomotic channels are identified can rational decisions concerning appropriate medical or surgical management be made. Techniques designed to evaluate the carotid artery bifurcation thus cannot provide definitive information, although they can identify those who may or may not need further evaluation.

From the therapeutic viewpoint, carotid, coronary, and intracranial arteriosclerosis must be considered together, because:

1. Many (though not all) of the risk factors are the same for each.

2. Arteriosclerosis in all these sites is very similar, and histopathological, cytopathological, and biochemical features of the lesions are, with very minor variations, the same.

3. Complicated lesions (thrombosis, stenosis, ectasia, plaque ulceration, and plaque hemorrhage) occur in all these sites, and even though their clinical expression depends on the vascular bed involved, their pathological process is the same in each.

4. Two-thirds of patients with intra- and extracranial arteriosclerosis succumb to myocardial infarction.

5. Postmortem examinations of Americans have shown that carotid and coronary artery arteriosclerosis become evident in the second decade of life and have a parallel evolution. This raises the possibility that examining the accessible extracranial carotid artery can give important clues to the state of coronary circulation.

Because the carotid bifurcation may be the most easily sampled segment of the arterial system, it is vital to develop methods to ascertain safely, reliably, and inexpensively the presence of asymptomatic lesions in this system in order to discern the presence of disease in less accessible arteries.

Since most stroke care is delivered in smaller hospitals, research and development programs are needed to perfect devices requiring minimal technical expertise for their accurate use and for the diagnostic interpretation of the data they produce. To prevent unguided proliferation of such equipment, unbiased testing of new models must be carried out in centers not involved in the original research and development, with appropriate studies to assess their sensitivity, specificity, reliability, and probable cost-benefit ratio in the health care system. Technical development must be encouraged by encouragement, not restriction, of inventiveness and innovation. Technology transfer should include support for demonstration centers and workshops for training biomedical scientists and clinical investigators.

One example of this is assessment of the ability of continuous-wave Doppler (CWD) ultrasound to reliably predict stenosis or occlusion at the carotid bifurcation. When the results of ultrasound testing were compared with those of cervical carotid arteriography in a study of 195 arteries of 105 patients with suspected carotid artery disease, Doppler alone was found to have no significant predictive value in arteries classified as from 0 to 50% stenosed. For stenoses greater than 50%, but not total, CWD was shown to predict the angiogram results with 70% reliability. The greatest correlation between the two methods was obtained in those arteries identified by CWD as being 75 to 95% stenosed. B-mode, OPG, and phonoangiography improve the sensitivity and specificity greatly.

These results indicate that much useful information can be obtained from noninvasive evaluation but that the arteriogram is superior overall. The importance of these studies must, nevertheless, be underscored, because noninvasive methods can identify individuals having a stenosis exceeding 50% with great reliability.

The authors in this volume considered the relative merits of the following modalities: X-ray, Doppler and B-mode ultrasound, positron emission transaxial tomograph (PETT) scanning, nuclear magnetic resonance (NMR), and physiologic methods of assessing pressure flow, pulse arrival, and contour. They agreed that, in the current state of the art, the two systems that give the most reliable information and appear to have the highest clinical potential are intravenous angiography and ultrasound.

Intravenous Angiography

Intravenous angiography has good potential for visualizing the entire intracranial arterial tree, but it cannot be used to assess lesions. With attainable improvements in its technology, it could be used to view all the arteries between the aortic arch and the brain. This system has yet to be evaluated fully, but it is apparently applicable to studies of asymptomatic patients with cervical murmurs, as well as symptomatic patients having had transient ischemic attacks.

Current State

This technique may be used to visualize all major arteries of the head, neck, thorax, abdomen, and extremities, as well as moderate to severe arterial lumen irregularities. It is a potential rival of direct angiography in detecting slight irregularities. Since it is more invasive than ultrasound, the latter should be the first choice to evaluate carotids, with intravenous angiography the first choice in all other areas.

Future Needs

1. Better and bigger intensifiers that can image a greater area of interest in detailed work.

2. Development and implementation of inexpensive mass storage media for images.

3. Design and development of injection catheters specific for this procedure.

4. Improved computer algorithms to increase the signal-to-noise contrast of arterial images and obtain quantitative morphological information.

5. Development of hard-copy recording techniques.

6. Improvement of video systems, especially their stability, dynamic range resolution, and noise characteristics.

7. Development of new X-ray contrast materials more suitable for this technique.

8. Development of X-ray tubes and generators with higher output capabilities.

9. Development of alternate detector systems.

10. Study of multienergy angiographic techniques.

It is important to realize that the X-ray characterizes the morphology but not the composition of the plaque. It may thus be useful in longitudinal studies of patients for the assessment of natural history and of medical and surgical interventions.

Ultrasound

Plaque Identification

With current instrumentation, ultrasound scans can identify some small lesions and most large ones. Some large lesions may be difficult to see because of loss of lumenal identification. Doppler systems probably are best for identifying medium and large lesions.

Characterization of the Lesion

Current systems can detect reflective and absorptive portions of a plaque but do not usually show the entire lesion, due to loss of detail, poor reflectivity, or shadowing caused by excess absorption. Doppler systems can show flow distortion.

The symptoms of lesions may be loosely correlated by ultrasound scanning to determine their size. The presence of a thrombus may be verified by finding a major change in lesion size. Doppler systems can reveal functional defects in a lesion, show the size of the lesion, and indicate surface characterization by recording flow disturbance patterns.

Future Needs

1. Ultrasound evaluation of the anatomical pathology and functional significance of lesions.

2. Spectral analysis of B-mode scans and of Doppler data to determine reflectivity, absorption, scattering, calcium content, lipid content, "soft plaque," and other physical or chemical properties of lesions.

3. Need to examine intracranial portion of carotid artery, as well as cervical portion. This means imaging through the intact adult skull.

4. Characterization of small lesions to determine content, morphology, relationship to wall layer, etc., to determine potential threat to health. Special effort is needed to identify thrombus formation in plaques.

Sizing of Lesions (Progression and Regression)

We must evaluate intervention measures for stabilizing lesions and promoting regression. Detectable and measurable features of lesions represent the best predictors of significant atherosclerosis leading to transient ischemic attacks. We must determine whether the severity of lesions in one vessel system corresponds with the severity of disease in another system. We must assess whether additional detail from B-scan images and Doppler flow patterns—parameters, such as lumen diameter, wall thickness, elasticity, and relative flow velocity—is of value. Improvements are needed in methods of assessing emerging systems for image reconstruction and interpretation, including three-dimensional displays and color coding of tissue characteristics and/or flow patterns.

With current technology, ultrasound scans can show the approximate size, shape, and location of a lesion, but cannot show the entire lesion. There is an estimated $\pm$ 20% error in detection of progression or regression of plaque when using existing systems. Doppler systems, however, can reveal any change in flow (which may accompany a change in size of a lesion), and the feasibility of this approach should be investigated. Neither system correlates well with thrombus or embolus, however.

Future Needs

1. Better resolution is needed in B-scans to allow smaller lesions to be seen.

2. Better Doppler flow measurements are needed to reduce background noise and eliminate effects of loss of signal due to intervening calcium.

3. B-scan and Doppler systems need to be integrated to take advantage of their complementary and supplementary features.

4. Precise measurement of lesion size may be important in assessing patients for possible surgery, perhaps eliminating the need for carotid angiography in selected patients. It is also important for use in intervention trials.

Rate of Change of the Process

With current technology, B-scan and Doppler methods can show rates of change if the lesions evolve within a specified time.

Future Needs

Faster regression of lesion size might result from specific drug interventions, diet modification, blood pressure control, surgery, and similar therapeutic modalities. Such attempts might be verified using B-scan, Doppler, or duplex systems with relative ease, reproducibility, and comfort to the patient, but improved systems are needed to make this practicable. Current systems are probably not suitable, due to their expense and large physical size and the need for improvements in their subsystems.

Detection of lesions and of functional changes in blood flow using B-scan Doppler equipment permits the physician to advise a patient on appropriate changes in lifestyle and the use of therapeutic drugs and to determine the need for angiography for diagnosis and for therapeutic surgery. Three-dimensional reconstruction techniques would also be useful in follow-up, since they are quickly interpretable, easily understandable, and conveniently stored.

It is essential that images of atherosclerotic arteries be validated using currently available ultrasound techniques. This includes acquisition of data, not only on arterial dimensions and tissue characteristics, but also on the relationship between these parameters and the functional state of the atherosclerotic artery. Such validation must not be limited to testing of the accuracy of measurements but must include assessment of the reproducibility of image generation and image interpretation, including estimates of intra- and interobserver variability. *In vivo* studies should be designed to compare and correlate data acquired noninvasively from angiographs and, when available, from surgical and autopsy specimens.

Morphological artifacts produced during surgical removal of endarterectomy specimens limit the value of dimensional data from such samples as compared with similar data obtained by other invasive or noninvasive methods. This calls for carefully controlled *in vitro* studies of excised human autopsy specimens, initially in static, and subsequently in pulsed-flow, systems, or combined *in vivo* and *in vitro* studies using animal models of atherosclerosis. In these types of studies, one can control precisely site identification, arterial pressure, and angles of interrogation.

Summary of Future Needs

Development of systems for the detection of plaques should include inprovement in ultrasonic technology to allow for the precise study of arterial wall morphology and assessment or progression and regression of lesions by noninvasive systems, both in human beings and animal models. There is a need to study plaque morphology, including tissue characterization and tissue "signature," using ultrasound. The following are needed: (a) an array echo-Doppler transducer; (b) real-time simultaneous tissue and flow imaging; (c) state-of-the-art resolution in Doppler techniques.

Nuclear Magnetic Resonance (NMR)

Although substances radioisotopes, such as 31^P, 13^C, and 23^{Na}, might be used to monitor more directly various physiological changes, their lower concentrations and weaker intrinsic signals would result in much lower resolutions or longer averaging times, even in very high magnetic fields. Such experiments are not yet practicable for most human diagnostic applications, although physiological studies of perfused organs in small animals may be possible. Attempts are being made to monitor cerebral ischemia and circulatory difficulties in the lower leg using very low-resolution 31^P NMR imaging.

Detecting Abnormalities, Pulse Contour, Arrival Time, and Pressure

The usefulness of data revealing arterial abnormalities, pulse contour, arrival time, and pressure is not known. Phonoangiographic recording of arterial murmurs and identification of changes in their characteristics over time are clinical skills that are just now being developed, and their practicality has yet to be assessed. Limited investigation of this seems justifiable.

Measurements of pressure, pulse contour, and arrival time within the ophthalmic arteries using a variety of instrumentation need to be compared with those taken using other technologies and bedside methods for direct assessment of the carotid and cerebral circulation. Such clinical correlations should be encouraged and should be followed by workshops and conferences to bring together investigators in this field to assess the state of the art.

ILIOFEMORAL ARTERY

Noninvasive diagnostic approaches to peripheral arterial occlusive disease entail many of the objectives and limitations detailed above for carotid artery disease. The clinical problems unique to peripheral arterial disease apply primarily to symptomatic patients; however, there is considerable justification for noninvasive detection of asymptomatic disease whether or not it is detectable by standard clinical examination. One precedent for this is the prospective screening of high-risk patients with diabetes mellitus using noninvasive physiological techniques. In the detection of clinically early disease, the most promising technique of identifying plaques is ultrasound.

Once asymptomatic disease is detected using physiological or ultrasonic techniques, confirmation of the presence, location, and extent of atherosclerotic plaque may one day be feasible using expected refinements in intravenous arteriography. However, a promising alternative for serial follow-up of the rate of change in plaque dimensions is high-resolution B-mode ultrasound, with its complementary velocity interrogation using real-time sound spectrum analysis of continuous or pulsed Doppler signals. Given the current state of the art, the peripheral arterial plaque location most accessible to instrumentation appears to be the bifurcation of the common femoral artery. As complementary methods of measuring the rate of progression or regression of asymptomatic or minimally symptomatic disease, physiological techniques employing segmental limb measurement of blood pressure, blood flow, and/or pulse wave analysis will continue to be helpful. Techniques for characterizing plaque constituents may be successful in peripheral arteries but are best validated in carotid lesions, which may be more accessible to noninvasive assessment and operative and pathological analysis.

Another aspect of the discussion concerning assessment of asymptomatic peripheral vascular disease was the need for intervention studies. Prospective clinical trials in high-risk groups, such as diabetes mellitus patients, might involve ultrasonic, intravenous angiographic, and physiological methods of endpoint analysis of disease progression or regression as adjuncts to such interventions as control of diabetes, cessation of cigarette smoking, and management of other risk factors.

The practice of noninvasive diagnosis and follow-up assessment in asymptomatic peripheral vascular disease appears fairly well defined. Patients presenting with symptoms of claudication, rest pain, or gangrene may be assessed using noninvasive techniques for the following purposes: (a) diagnostic confirmation; (b) anatomic localization; (c) determination of physiological impairment; (d) selection of therapy (medical, balloon dilatation, operative reconstruction); (e) monitoring of therapeutic intervention (intraoperative and postoperative monitoring, prediction of therapeutic result); and (f) late serial follow-up.

The various physiological and noninvasive techniques provide both qualitative and quantitative information in all of these areas.

Intravenous arteriography—so-called digital radiography—seems the most suitable noninvasive method for morphological confirmation of symptomatic peripheral arterial occlusive disease in patients who are candidates for operation. Current techniques are limited by their relatively small field of view, considering the wide extent of disease to be visualized in most symptomatic patients. Refiners of image-enhancing systems must consider that patients with lower extremity symptoms who may be candidates for operation must be assessed across the entire arterial tree, from the infrarenal abdominal aorta to the distal tibial arteries. High-resolution imaging of plaques, however, will not be necessary.

Current instrumentation provides a contrast resolution that allows detection of plaques of moderate clinical activity, although it overlooks subtle wall disease. Its submillimeter spatial and temporal resolution are more than adequate. Low-cost image storage media and an improved injection technique are needed, however, and that technique must provide sufficient contrast enhancement to detect patency of specific major arteries that might be involved in arterial reconstruction. Ultrasonic techniques currently seem ill suited for such extensive vascular analysis.

Future Needs

The foregoing discussion assumes that the ultrasonic and intravenous radiologic techniques in question will have been appropriately validated. Their sensitivity, specificity, and reproducibility are best assessed in the carotid arterial system, *in vitro*, or in models. Intravenous arteriography may, in fact, be most appropriately validated in candidates for operative therapy, who normally undergo contrast arteriography. The physiological techniques for this procedure have been used for a number of years, and most were validated before their introduction. Physicians developing noninvasive peripheral vascular laboratories are being taught these skills. The objectives of such technology transfer must, indeed, include programs of training for physicians and technologists, in both the appropriate application and the interpretation of results from these established methods.

The future of the more complex techniques of nuclear magnetic resonance and PETT in combating clinical peripheral vascular disease is unclear. Although they may eventually be used to provide estimates of volume blood flow in peripheral tissues, such information will have limited clinical application in any but the most advanced states of arterial insufficiency—which, in any case, are more readily assessed using less complex techniques. A more realistic product of these investigative techniques may be the information they provide about tissue characteristics and biochemical activity. The potential clinical uses of such results, however, remain to be defined.

Noninvasive Techniques for Assessment of Atherosclerosis in Peripheral, Carotid, and Coronary Arteries, edited by Thomas F. Budinger, et al. Raven Press, New York 1982.

Concluding Statement

Richard S. Ross

Department of Medicine, Johns Hopkins University School of Medicine, Baltimore, Maryland 21218

The characteristics of the atherosclerotic lesion were stressed because of the importance of this subject to the detection of the lesion *in vivo*. The lesion is a mixture of fibrous, lipid, and other tissues, and calcium is often present. Layers of foam cells and platelets have been visualized by scanning electron microscopy on the surface of the vessel wall. The composition of the lesion is important only as a clue to various techniques for imaging or labeling. If specialists know what is in the plaque, they will be better able to look for it. The composition is also important with respect to the susceptibility of the lesion to dilatation techniques, such as percutaneous transluminal coronary angioplasty.

It was pointed out that the atherosclerotic lesion is located within the wall of the artery and that the lumen is round or elliptical in the living state. The common histological picture, which shows the encroachment of the atheroma into the lumen, is probably an artifact of the fixation.

ASYMPTOMATIC PERIPHERAL AND CAROTID ARTERIES

These minimal lesions can usually be detected by ultrasound imaging, the Doppler technique, or a combination of the two. Correlation between these noninvasive techniques and arteriography or pathological material has been made in the severe symptomatic disease states, but not in minimal disease so far.

PERIPHERAL SYMPTOMATIC

The best way of evaluating symptomatic peripheral disease is probably by functional tests of blood flow, especially during stress—as with exercise, for example. Other useful techniques involve the differential measurement of blood pressure in the leg.

SYMPTOMATIC CAROTID

The angiogram is currently the best method of detecting lesions in the carotid system. Especially encouraging in this regard is the new work using right-sided injections with contrast material and image enhancement. Of the noninvasive methods, B-scan ultrasound, especially when combined with Doppler, appears to have great potential.

CORONARY ARTERIES

The coronaries present an especially difficult problem because they are small, deep in the chest, and are moving. Currently, virtually all specialists agree that the only satisfactory way of getting anatomic information about the coronary arteries is with high quality selective coronary arteriography. It is possible to visualize coronary arteries by ultrasound, especially the large proximal segments.

It is also possible to see coronary arteries by intravenous injections with subtraction image enhancement, but the quality necessary for intervention or for the quantitation of the plaque is probably not available with any technique other than arteriography. It would seem appropriate to proceed with noninvasive techniques for the larger, more easily visualized vessels, such as the carotid and peripheral vessels, with application to the coronaries to come later.

As to future directions, the following suggestions seem pertinent:

1. There is need for more information about the physical characteristics of the tissue in the atherosclerotic plaque. This is not meant to imply clinical analysis of plaque but rather of the absorption properties of the material with regard to X-rays, especially monoenergetic sources. It is important to know something about the metabolism of the plaque. Both positron emission transaxial tomography and nuclear magnetic resonance techniques may be applicable in this regard in the future.

2. The concept of the risk/benefit ratio should be introduced into the considerations. Certain invasive studies may be necessary if they can provide much better information. We should not be obsessed with the necessity of totally noninvasive studies if, for example, a right heart injection is far superior to a peripheral venous injection for right-sided angiography.

3. There is a need for additional studies of the effects of ultrasonic energy on tissue, especially platelets, endothelium, and DNA strands. Although there is no evidence that ultrasound is damaging to tissue, this possibility deserves careful investigation.

4. There is a need for a critical examination of the magnitude of change that might be expected in atherosclerotic vessels. We need to know how much change we can expect in the regression and progression of atherosclerotic disease in human patients. This needs to be assessed under ideal conditions with good quantitative angiography. When we know how major these changes are, then we will know what level of sensitivity is required for noninvasive studies. There is still a real question as to whether the permanent, fully developed atherosclerotic plaque can regress. Some of the so-called regression changes that we identify may actually be the result of the disappearance of a platelet clot.

Many specialists consider angiography to be the "gold standard," but it is quite apparent that there are errors in angiography that need to be assessed. Observer error from day to day or from observer to observer is one thing, but the other, less easily controlled variable is that having to do with physiological variability in the patient from day to day. It must be recognized that vascular tone, hemodynamic status, cardiac output, and the development of collateral circulation with alternate blood flow pathways may all alter the patient's angiographic appearance.

Subject Index